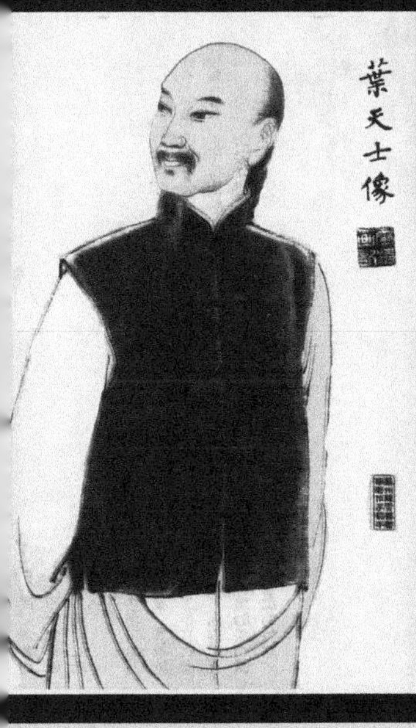

Translated by

JIAN MIN WEN

and

GARRY SEIFERT

Warm Disease Theory

Wēn Bìng Xué

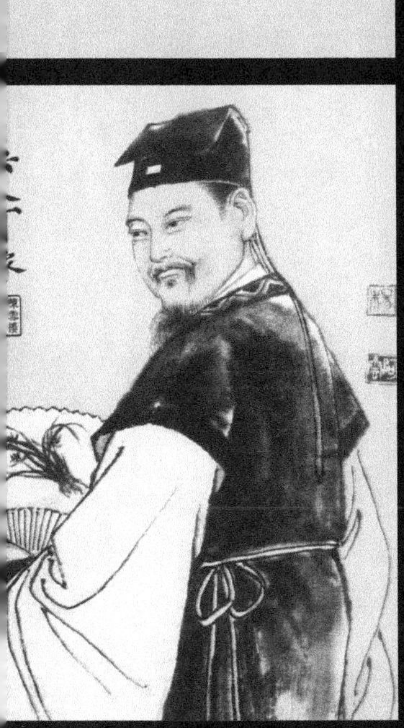

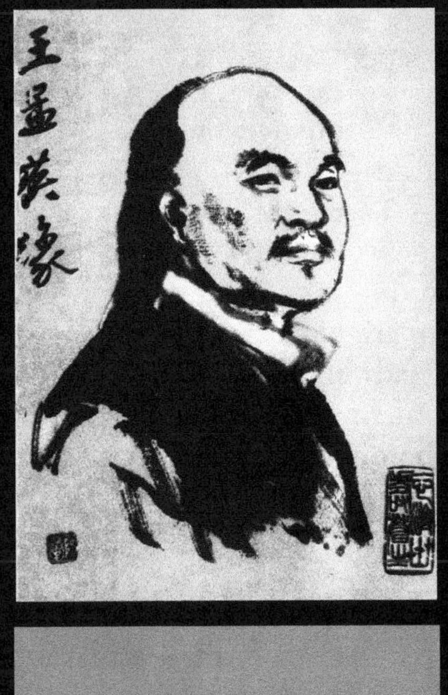

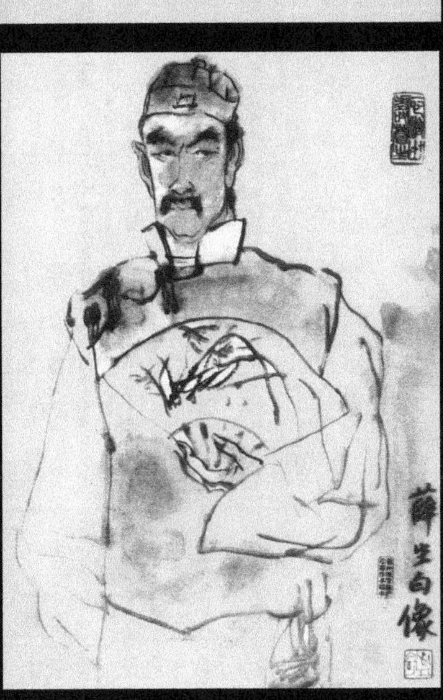

WARM DISEASE THEORY
WĒN BÌNG XUÉ

Translated by
Jian Min Wen and Garry Seifert

ISBN 0-912111-74-7

Library of Congress Cataloging-In-Publication Data:

Wen ping hsèueh. English.
Warm disease theory : Wen bing xue / translated by Jian Min Wen and Garry Seifert.
p. cm.
Translation of: Wen bing xue.
ISBN 0-912111-61-5
1. Medicine, Chinese. I. Title: Wen bing xue. II. Wen, Jian Min. III. Seifert, Garry. IV. Title.
R602 .W3413 2000
610'.951--dc21
00-010622

~Published by ~
Paradigm Publications
Taos, NM, USA
http://www.paradigm-pubs.com
Printed in the United States of America

CONTENTS

FOREWORD

This book is based on a translation extracted from the standard warm disease text used by all Chinese Institutes of Chinese Medicine.

Although there were several schools of warm disease, dating from the Míng (明) and Qīng (清) dynasties, until the time this text was written there had never been an attempt to integrate their ideas into an overview. Even the great Míng and Qīng Dynasty doctors of warm disease, on whose works this text is based, only had partial insights—their views were relatively fragmentary. This is the first text to integrate the views of every school, the first to undertake a comprehensive discussion of the foundations of warm disease theory and the clinical treatment of warm diseases. It is in fact such a valuable source of theoretical and therapeutic information that it is often considered a modern classic.

The work is arranged in two sections. The first introduces all the basic information about warm disease, including its history, disease causes, pattern identification, and general diagnostic and treatment methods. The second section devotes a separate chapter to each of the different warm diseases. It deals with the disease factors, clinical manifestations, pulses and treatments in the warm diseases of the four seasons including wind warmth, spring warmth, summerheat warmth, damp warmth, latent summerheat warmth, autumn dryness, and warm toxins. In each of these warm diseases, the disease concepts, etiologies, pathologies, main points of diagnosis and treatment policies are discussed first, then the patterns and treatments of their characteristic disease transformations are explained.

TRANSLATORS' PREFACE

This book is called *Warm Disease Theory*, which is our translation of the term "*Wēn Bìng Xué*" (溫病學). "Warm disease" is a literal translation. It has exactly the same connotations in English as *wēn bìng* has in Chinese. We decided not to adopt the other common translation, "febrile disease," because the idea behind this usage seems to be that the term *wēn* is actually a metaphor for fever. Although exuberant fever is usually the main symptom in warm disease, there are certain patterns such as dampness winning and *yáng* weakening in damp warmth diseases where fever does not occur at all. It is our belief that because "warm disease" does not have a pre-existing specific technical meaning, it is a better translation.

Most of the technical terms in this book have been adopted from the Paradigm Publications house standard (i.e., from the Wiseman system of translation). Prior to the creation of this standard, there was a pronounced tendency for every different translator or author of Chinese medicine texts to translate same terminologies in different ways, so it was seldom clear whether different authors were talking about the same concepts or subtly different concepts. This made it virtually impossible for students to properly cross-reference material, and therefore also made it very difficult for them to properly understand the various subjects of their studies.

Adopting a house standard is a sensible way for publishing companies such as Paradigm to address this problem. The Wiseman standard is based on well-documented rationales and has a well-planned style. It is therefore a good standard, particularly for those who are studying not only Chinese medicine, but also the Chinese language of Chinese medicine.

For the sake of helping to provide students with a relatively uniform set of texts, we have seldom deviated from this standard. We have only done so on the rare occasions where we have considered it possible to clarify the meaning intended by the original Chinese, or to make text easier to understand in other ways. All such changes are listed in the Glossary of Uncommon Chinese Medical Terms at the end of the book.

We are aware that the Wiseman system has its critics. Mr. Wiseman's desire to enable readers to trace back from a translation to its source language insinuates a generalist approach. Instead of translating a single word or term differently in different contexts, he always tends to translate words in the same way. Where plausible he always tries to find an English language word that conveys all possible meanings of the original Chinese. This strategy makes it relatively easy to link translated words with source-language words, and thereby facilitates the study of Chinese language. However, it does not necessarily facilitate a concise, clinically oriented understanding of word meaning in context—the reason being that words tend to take on specific meanings according to the contexts in which they are used, and generalist translations do not always convey these specific meanings. Most Western criticisms of the Wiseman system appear to stem from this weakness.

Whether one believes this weakness to be significant or not, it is fair to say that the Wiseman standard has not been universally embraced. The acceptability or unacceptability of a translation or a translation system ultimately depends on the perspectives of its users. Perspectives are formed not only for academic reasons but also for historical, political, and social reasons. Without adequate communications it is nearly impossible for the perspectives held by any one school of thought to be fully understood by any other because practical circumstances vary so greatly.

We believe that the best way to create a more universally acceptable translation system would be to establish an international forum consisting of people who have a good understanding of Chinese medical theory and a rich experience in clinical practice, people who understand ancient Chinese languages, people who understand English and translating methods, and people who understand biomedicine.

Finally, we should like to add a word on inconsistencies between formula text and formula commentaries. In the original Chinese text on which this work is based herbs are not always given the same names in formulas as in the commentaries that follow.

There are three reasons for this. Firstly, herb names are commonly abbreviated. For example, raw licorice root (*shēng gān cǎo*) listed in a formula, becomes licorice root (*gān cǎo*) discussed in its commentary. Secondly, herb names are sometimes expanded. For example, gardenia [fruit] (*zhī zǐ*) listed in a formula, becomes gardenia [fruit] (*shān zhī zǐ*) discussed in its commentary. And thirdly, herb names are occasionally adjusted or named more fully to make their identification easier. For example peony (*sháo yào*) listed in a formula, becomes white peony (*bái sháo*) discussed in its commentary. These types of inconsistencies are extensive but not confusing.

Another type of inconsistency is that herbs are sometimes omitted either from formulas or the commentaries that follow. Often instead of being listed in formulas, fresh herbs (which are difficult to store and therefore to dispense) or ingredients that might be considered additives form a Western perspective are not listed in formulas but introduced in formula preparation, and then discussed in formula commentary. Sometimes herbs listed in formulas are not discussed in commentaries, and sometimes when herbs are discussed in commentaries, instructions are given to omit them. The reasons for these kinds of inconsistency are unclear, but we do not believe they detract from the text so we have made no attempt to adjust them.

Prof. Jian Min Wen 温健民
China Academy of Traditional Chinese Medicine, Beijing, China

Garry Seifert
Lifegate College of Traditional Chinese Medicine, Sydney, Australia

August, 2000

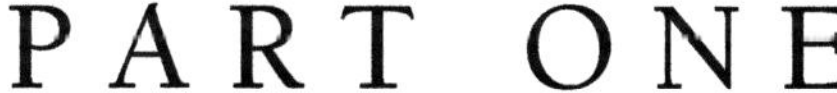

PART ONE

INTRODUCTION

In Chinese medicine there are four classics that all serious students are required to study. These include the *Classic of Internal Medicine* (*Nèi Jīng* 內經), *Treatise on Cold Damage* (*Shāng Hán Lùn* 傷寒論), *Synopsis of the Golden Chamber* (*Jīn Kuì Yào Luè* 金匱要略), and *Warm Disease Theory* (*Wēn Bìng Xué* 溫病學).

The *Classic of Internal Medicine* is the oldest and greatest of these four classics. Although ascribed to the Yellow Emperor (Huáng Dì 黃帝), it was actually written during the Warring States Period (475 B.C.–221 B.C.) by numerous unknown authors. It consists of two parts: the *Plain Questions* (*Sù Wèn* 素問) and the *Miraculous Pivot* (*Lìng Shū* 靈樞).

Originally, the *Plain Questions* had nine volumes and 81 articles. Of these, only eight volumes survived the Wèi Jìn (魏晉) Period. During the Táng (唐) Dynasty these were divided into 24 volumes by Wáng Bīng (王冰) who not only added notes and commentaries but also wrote replacements for some of the lost articles. Later, in the Nán Sòng (南宋) Dynasty, Lín Yì (林億) checked the text anew and added more notes. His work became the basis for all subsequent editions. Some of the main subjects in the *Plain Questions* include anatomy, physiology, pathogens, pathology, diagnosis, pattern differentiation, treatment, disease prevention, health preservation, relationships between man and nature, applications of *yīn-yáng* and five phase theory in medicine, and *qì* flow theory.

The *Miraculous Pivot* contains similar subject matter to the *Plain Questions,* but deals less with the circulatory movements through the five phases and more with the channels and the needling of points.

The *Treatise on Cold Damage and Miscellaneous Diseases* (*Shāng Hán Zá Bìng Lùn* 傷寒雜病論) was written by Zhāng Zhòng Jǐng (張仲景) in the Dōng Hàn (東漢) Dynasty. About one hundred years later, in the Jìn (晉) Dynasty, it was rearranged in two separate texts by Wáng Shū Hé (王叔和). One text consisted of ten volumes and was called the *Treatise on Cold Damage* (*Shāng Hán Lùn* 傷寒論); the other consisted of three volumes and was called the *Synopsis of the Golden Chamber* (*Jīn Kuì Yào Luè* 金匱要略). Subsequently, in the Sòng (宋) Dynasty, these texts were rearranged by the Bureau for Editing and Publishing Medical Books.

The *Treatise on Cold Damage* analyzes and differentiates externally contracted diseases according to six-channel theory. The *Synopsis of the Golden Chamber* deals mainly with the miscellaneous diseases of internal medicine, but also touches on external and women's diseases.

Warm Disease Theory (*Wēn Bìng Xué* 溫病學) is the most modern of the four classics. In this context, the term "classic" means an area of classical study rather than a single classical text. Even though there are numerous references to warm diseases in very ancient texts, warm disease was not developed as an independent system until the Qīng (清) Dynasty. The five medical experts whose influences were most instrumental in facilitating this process were Wú Yòu Kě (吳又可), Yè Tiān Shì (葉天士), Xuē Shēng Bái (薛生白), Wú Jú Tōng (吳鞠通), and Wáng Mèng Yīng (王孟英). The first of these, Wú Yòu Kě, lived in the Míng Dynasty. The other four medical experts all lived during the Qīng Dynasty.

Wú Jú Tōng put forward the theory of pestilence *qì* (*lì qì* 戾氣) to explicate the role of certain infectious factors in the etiology of communicable diseases. His was the first theory to assert that warm pathogens enter the body through the mouth and nose. He published these ideas in his *Treatise on Acute Epidemic Warmth* (*Wēn Yì Lùn* 溫疫論).

Yè Tiān Shì introduced the theory that warm diseases develop and transmit through four aspects—namely the defense, *qì*, construction, and blood aspects. His lectures and teachings were edited by his disciples and published in the *Treatise on Warm Heat* (*Wēn Rè Lùn* 溫熱論).

Xuē Shēng Bái concentrated on discussing damp-heat disease factors. He clearly explained that damp-heat usually occurs from a combination of external *yáng* brightness and internal greater *yīn* factors affecting each other. He published his ideas in his *Detailed Analysis of Damp-Heat* (*Shī Rè Tiáo Biàn* 濕熱條辯).

Wú Jú Tōng expanded on the ideas of Dr Yè Tiān Shì by developing a system of differential diagnosis based on the pathological changes in the triple burner. He summarized his findings and published them in his *Detailed Analysis of Warm Diseases* (*Wēn Bìng Tiáo Biàn* 溫病條辯).

Wáng Mèng Yīng developed insights on the cause of warm fevers, their symptoms, and their treatment methods, by applying the theories set down in the *Classic of Internal Medicine* and *Treatise on Cold Damage* to the views of his renowned contemporaries. He published his ideas in several books, the most important of which is *Warm Heat Latitudes and Longitudes* (*Wēn Rè Jīng Wěi* 温热经纬).

Based on the different theories and practices of cold damage and warm disease, two contending schools of medical thought arose. Medical practitioners who followed the theories as set out in the *Treatise on Cold Damage* were said to belong to the cold damage school, whereas practitioners who followed warm disease theories were said to belong to the warm disease school. Although both these schools held certain common principles, there were also many differences between them. From the beginning of the Qīng Dynasty, the medical experts of both schools debated the value of warm disease and the relationship between warm disease and cold damage.

Members of the cold damage school argued that cold damage referred to all externally contracted hot diseases, including warm diseases. They accepted that the *Treatise on Cold Damage* had not proposed any clear methods for treating warm diseases, but pointed out that the *yáng* brightness disease pattern was actually a clinical manifestation of warm disease, and that both White Tiger Decoction (*Bái Hǔ Tāng*) and Qì-Infusing Decoction (*Chéng Qì Tāng*) were actually warm disease formulas. Consequently, they were of the opinion that Zhāng Zhòng Jǐng's book dealt with all externally contracted diseases (not only externally contracted wind-cold), and that six-channel theory could therefore be suitably applied in warm diseases. Based on this view, numerous prominent physicians of the cold disease school argued that there was no need to separate warm disease from cold damage.

The warm disease school, on the other hand, held the view that warm diseases and cold damage were two different types of externally contracted diseases, with different treatments and different concepts. They reasoned that even though the *Treatise on Cold Damage* was a book that dealt specifically with externally contracted diseases, it was detailed in regard to cold but sketchy in regard to warmth. In the chapter on greater *yáng* disease, for instance, warm diseases are mentioned but clear treatment methods are not recommended, yet for cold diseases and wind stroke there are detailed discussions and treatments. Also, even though White Tiger Decoction and Qì-Infusing Decoction can be used in warm diseases, they are not suitable for use throughout the whole disease process. Therefore, the medical experts of the warm disease school had strong convictions that warm disease must be established as an independent system.

The first theories on the treatment of externally contracted hot diseases were set out in the *Treatise on Cold Damage*, and after a long period of development, the theories of warm disease were the next major step. In regard to the special area of externally contracted warm diseases, the ideas in *Warm Disease Theory* are more effective than those in the *Treatise on Cold Damage*. Often, warm disease theories supplement cold damage theories and enhance their clinical effectiveness. Therefore, once the warm disease theories took form, they quickly spread throughout all China and were embraced by most medical practitioners.

Thus the *Treatise on Cold Damage* made a significant contribution towards the treatment of hot disease, in that to some extent, the development of the warm disease school was based on the cold damage school's policies of pattern differentiation and treatment identification. In fact, some of the treatment methods which the warm disease school adopted from the cold damage school are valuable in clinical practice even today. Nevertheless, because of technological limitations in the Dōng Hàn Dynasty when it was originally completed, the *Treatise on Cold Damage* was unable to explain certain types of warm disease.

As technology developed and medical experts accumulated more experience, practitioners of Chinese medicine cultivated and advanced their technical knowledge. Using the theories in the *Treatise on Cold Damage* as a basis, they summarized their clinical experiences and developed new theories and treatment methods that were suitable for their own times. In short, from cold damage to warm disease is a continuous, unbroken line of knowledge. The *Treatise on Cold Damage* is the foundation of the *Warm Disease Theory,* and the *Warm Disease Theory* supplements the *Treatise on Cold Damage.* Of course, even *Warm Disease Theory* has its limitations and must be improved further in the future.

Three of the above classics—the *Classic of Internal Medicine*, the *Treatise on Cold Damage,* and the *Synopsis of the Golden Chamber*—have already been translated into English. Until now, *Warm Disease Theory* has not. As already stated, *Warm Disease Theory* includes the ideas of several medical experts, but actually each of these experts only had a limited understanding; none of them had a complete picture, so none of their views can be considered representative of the whole system.

In introducing *Warm Disease Theory* to the West, we have carefully selected a text that will present the entire system as an integrated whole. Selecting one of the older texts would only have led to an unbalanced, partial view. By studying this work, and developing an understanding of its content, it becomes relatively easy to study the more ancient texts at a later date.

The text we have selected is the standard text used by all institutes of Chinese medicine, throughout China. The original Chinese version was commissioned by the Ministry of Health and Higher Education, edited under the supervision of Mèng Shù Jiāng (孟澍江), Shěn Fèng Gé (沈鳳閣), Wáng Càn Huī (王燦輝) and Yù Jué Chū (鬱覺初) through the Nán Jīng College of Traditional Chinese Medicine. It was first published in 1979 by Research and Technical Publications of Shanghai, and from that time has been a compulsory text in all training institutions from which graduate students become registered doctors of Traditional Chinese Medicine.

In China, if you wish to become a registered doctor of Traditional Chinese medicine, there are two paths open to you. You may either study as an apprentice, at the side of an established practitioner, or you must pass the national entrance examination at an institute of Traditional Chinese Medicine. In the former case, at the end of your apprenticeship you must sit the national exam; if you pass you are registered. In the latter case, you will be automatically registered when you pass your final-year exam.

No matter which of these paths you take, you must study the same basic subjects, although in the institutes you also need to study additional subjects, most of which relate to modern biomedicine. There are about 20 subjects common to both pathways—the number varies from year to year. Training in the institutes is, however, organized in a more systematic way. Before studying warm disease, students must first study the fundamental theories of Chinese medicine, Chinese medicine medicinal substances, Chinese medicine prescriptions, and the *Classic of Internal Medicine*. They do not study *Warm Disease Theory* until some time in their second year. Warm disease is taught over approximately 100 hours of lectures.

It may also be of interest to note that the structure of a full five- or six-year course in China is quite different from the structure of a bachelor's degree course in the West. In China the first four years are spent studying in an institute; the last year is spent studying in a hospital. About 42 weeks a year are spent on campus—six days a week, eight hours a day. After finishing their internships, graduates becomes registered bachelors of Chinese medicine. At this time they can choose to enter clinical practice or to continue studying. Those who decide to continue studying must first select a subject, pass an entrance exam on that subject, then concentrate on studying theory in a single area of special interest for another three years. After that, if they pass an exam, Master's Degrees of Theory are awarded.

If bachelor's degree graduates choose to enter clinical practice, after two years, they may resume their studies, and if they then pass an entrance exam, may work on a practical master's degree, which takes another three years to complete. Once students have a master's degree, if they pass another entrance exam, they may study for a Ph.D., which takes another two or three years. After this, if they pass their exams, they are awarded a Ph.D. Warm disease is one of the special subjects that can be studied at both the master and Ph.D. levels. This *Warm Disease Theory* text is still used at all these levels, but deeper research is also required.

Traditional Chinese Medicine was introduced into institutions of advanced education in 1957. But the current system of education was not established until 1977 and the first bachelor's degrees were not awarded until 1983.

CHAPTER 1

WARM DISEASE DEVELOPMENT AND HISTORY

Warm disease is one of the many clinical subjects of Chinese medicine. It expounds on the warm diseases of the four seasons, covering the rationale behind their occurrence and development, and also their diagnosis and treatment, with two main aims. The first is to divulge the nature of warm diseases by clearly explaining the reasons for their occurrence, the disposition of their pathological changes, and the laws that govern their transformations and alterations. The second is to progress on this basis into the study and discussion of warm disease diagnostic methods and treatment measures so that effective therapeutic results may be achieved.

Since warm diseases are still very commonly seen in contemporary clinical practices, and since they occur throughout all four seasons of the year, affecting males, females, old and young alike, the warm disease system is one of the most important practical subjects in Chinese medicine. Warm diseases usually occur with rapid onset and development, have severe ramifications, and are, in most cases, infectious; sometimes, under certain conditions, they can even give rise to epidemics. It is therefore important to implement a policy of prevention. Using appropriate prevention methods is the best way to keep the incidence of these diseases under control.

The warm disease system has a long history of development. Since there are many ways in which the characteristics of warm diseases are different from other diseases, it took the medical experts of ancient times long periods of clinical observation and practical experience to recognize their basic laws and, little by little, to encapsulate these into the theory of stratagems and methods of diagnosis and treatment currently called the warm disease system. The steps by which this system took form are related below.

I. RUDIMENTARY BEGINNINGS

The rudimentary step in the formation of the warm disease system took place during the Warring States (Zhàn Guó 戰國) Period, and through the Qín (秦), Hàn (漢), Jìn (晉), and Táng (唐) Dynasties (i.e., from 255 BC to 907 AD). Although there are no specific discussions on warm disease in any of the medical records of these periods, there are certain mentions of pathomechanisms, patterns, pulses, and treatments.

The *Classic of Internal Medicine* mentions warm disease victims and warm disease outbreaks and these are the earliest uses of warm disease as a term. Expounding on pathomechanisms, it also mentions that damage by cold in winter must lead to warm diseases during spring. This introduces the rudimentary theory on which later generations based their views about the latent pathomechanism of warm diseases. The most typical Hàn Dynasty discussions can be found in Zhāng Zhòng Jǐng's *Treatise on Cold Damage*. In regard to symptoms, one passage says, "Greater *yáng* diseases with fever and thirst but no aversion to cold indicate warm disease."

Although very simple, this extract clearly states that at the beginning of a warm disease, hot signs are stronger than cold. On treatment, the *Classic of Internal Medicine* established the policy that "heat should be cooled." This is the earliest rudimentary theory about warm disease treatment. Although the *Treatise on Cold Damage* gave no indications as to the use of formulas for the management of warm diseases, it did describe the heat-clearing and downward-throughclearing methods, both of which are effective warm disease treatments. When subsequent generations developed warm disease treatment methods, these ideas had a profound influence. Later, in the Táng Dynasty, Chinese medical books like *Prescriptions Worth a Thousand Pieces of Gold (Qiān Jīn Fāng 千金方)* and *Medical Secrets of an Official (Wài Tái Mì Yào 外臺秘要)* also described several formulas dealing with the prevention and treatment of warm diseases. For example, the smoke of Supreme Unity Flowing Gold Powder *(Tài Yī Liú Jīn Sǎn 太乙流金散)* was used to prevent warm diseases, Solomon's Seal [Root] Decoction *(Wěi Ruí Tāng 萎蕤湯)* was used to treat wind warmth, and Black Paste Decoction *(Hēi Gāo Tāng 黑膏湯)* was used to treat warm toxins surfacing as macula. All the above treatments still have a certain clinical relevance.

In short, although warm diseases were partially understood before the Táng Dynasty, theory was still rudimentary. Warm disease and cold damage concepts were not very clearly distinguished. Warm diseases were still classed as cold damage. The *Classic of Internal Medicine,* for instance, declared:

> *All hot diseases belong to the category of cold damage. ... If a patient is suffering from cold damage, later warmth can develop. Before summer, these diseases are called warm [diseases]; after summer they are called summerheat diseases.*

Later, based on this theory, the *Classic on Medical Problems* (*Nàn Jīng* 難經) divided cold damage into five disease pattern subcategories: wind stroke, cold damage, damp warmth, hot disease, and wind disease. Clearly, at this time, warm diseases were considered a type of cold damage.

II. THE DEVELOPMENTAL STAGE

The developmental stage in the formation of the warm disease system took place from the Sòng (宋) Dynasty through to the end of the Jīn Yuán (金元) Dynasty (960 AD. to 1368 AD.). During this stage, there were breakthroughs regarding the logic, methods, prescriptions, and medicinals for treating warm diseases—particularly the methods for their treatment. This enabled warm disease theory to start developing as a separate system.

In the centuries after Zhāng Zhòng Jǐng adopted the concepts outlined in the *Classic of Internal Medicine* as a basis for organizing his *Treatise on Cold Damage* and establishing a differentiation and treatment system for externally contracted diseases, the logic and treatment methods, prescriptions and medicinals of the *Treatise on Cold Damage* were adopted as a general standard for the basic management of all externally contracted diseases. However, as society evolved and medical practice grew in scope, the shortcomings of the *Treatise on Cold Damage* treatment system became obvious—it needed development and expansion. Accordingly, from the beginning of the Sòng Dynasty, numerous different medical experts began, one after the other, to advocate their various opinions on augmenting and reforming the established methods for treating externally contracted hot diseases.

Zhū Gōng (朱肱) of the Sòng Dynasty, for instance, was first to advance the view that the acrid warm outthrusting formulas from the *Treatise on Cold Damage,* such as Ephedra Decoction (*Má Huáng Tāng* 麻黃湯) and Cinnamon Twig Decoction (*Guì Zhī Tāng* 桂枝湯), should be adjusted prior to prescription in order to suit the clinical situation as influenced by the time, the place, and the patient's condition. This opinion contributed to the development of medicine by challenging the established medical dogma of his era—that *Treatise on Cold Damage* formulas be used without modification. During the Jìn Dynasty many different schools of contending medical interpretations arose. These acted as a powerful catalyst for the development of warm disease theory, particularly in the area of treatment.

Exemplifying the revolutionary ideas put forward at that time was the assertion that ancient formulas were no longer appropriate for modern diseases. Liú Hé Jiān (劉河間), for instance (one of the four famous Jìn Yuán Dynasty medical experts), advocated bold new ideas, treatment methods, and formulas for the management of hot diseases. Later, these were acknowledged as important contributions to the advancement and development of warm disease treatment methods.

On the basis of his clinical experiences, Liú Hé Jiān concluded that all six-channel transformations discussed in the *Treatise on Cold Damage* were actually attributable to hot patterns, and that they must therefore all be treated principally with cold and cooling medicinals.

He also stressed the inappropriateness of using only acrid, warm exterior-resolving methods during the initial stages of hot diseases. He pointed out that the hotter acrid warming prescriptions, based on combinations of medicinals such as ephedra (*má huáng*) and cinnamon twig (*guì zhī*), could easily cause severe adverse reactions, and he recommended that the acrid cooling method be used instead, so as to resolve the exterior and interior simultaneously. Accordingly, he developed prescriptions like Double-Resolution Powder (*Shuāng Jiě Săn* 雙解散) and Diaphragm-Cooling Powder (*Liáng Gé Săn* 涼膈散). His theory on the use of cold and cool heat-clearing medicinals as the main treatment system for warm diseases set future generations on a clear path and marked a major change of direction in warm disease history. His successors therefore said, "For cold damage follow the ideas of Zhāng Zhòng Jǐng; for hot diseases follow the ideas of Hé Jiān."

Towards the end of the Yuán Dynasty, the medical expert Wáng Ān Dào (王安道) clearly differentiated the concepts, pathomechanisms, and treatments of warm diseases and cold damage. He pointed out that warm diseases should not be confused with cold damage; in warm diseases, the pathomechanism is latent heat emerging from interior to exterior, so the principal treatment must be to clear the internal heat. From then on, physicians began to distinguish warm diseases from cold injuries. For this reason, the Qīng Dynasty warm disease medical expert Wú Jú Tōng (吳鞠通) commended Wáng Ān Dào for differentiating and beginning to distinguish warm diseases from cold damage.

III. THE FORMATIVE STAGE

Throughout the Míng Dynasty (1368 to 1644 AD) and Qīng Dynasty (1644 AD to 1911 AD), warm disease theory underwent maturation. The thinking deepened, the theory became more and more perfected, and the treatments grew richer and richer. The ideological constructs were condensed into a more complete system of theories and methods for warm disease pattern identification and treatment determination, and a single system of logic, treatment methods, prescriptions, and medicinals emerged.

Wāng Shí Shān (汪石山), a Míng Dynasty medical expert, advanced a very clear idea concerning newly contracted warm disease. It was his view that warm diseases were caused not only by latent warm disease pathogens ("damage by cold in winter that must come out during spring"), but also by newly contracted warm disease pathogens ("not damage by cold in winter"). This broke from traditional ideas about latent pathogens transforming into heat.

During the latter stages of the Míng Dynasty another medical expert, Wú Yòu Kě (吳又可), working with the learning and experiences of previous generations, developed his own empirical theories, and on this basis compiled the *Treatise on Acute Epidemic Warmth* (*Wēn Yì Lùn* 溫疫論), the first book that specialized in warm disease theory. In this work, he put forward several original views about the differences between warm pestilence diseases and cold damage diseases. For example, in regard to pathomechanics, he asserted that epidemic warm diseases are caused not only by the six pathogenic *qì* of wind, cold, summerheat, heat, dryness, and dampness, but also by a peculiar substance of the natural world called pestilential *qì*. In regard to epidemiology, he declared that warm pestilential diseases have a strongly infectious nature, "transferring by touch to old and young alike," and that infections occur via the mouth and nose. In regard to therapy, he pointed out that the first priority of treatment should be to dispel pathogens with coursing, disinhibiting, and outthrusting methods. These opinions, which were at that time completely original, are still very useful even today.

During the Qīng Dynasty, both the defense-*qì*-construction-blood concept and the triple burner concept were developed to form a single complete system of warm disease etiologies, patterns, pulses, and treatments. By this time, the application of warm disease theory was already widespread in southern China. Subsequently, several medical experts including Yè Tiān Shì, Xuē Shēng Bái, Wú Jú Tōng, and Wáng Mèng Yīng arose. Their bold ideas broke away from the traditional views that "warm diseases never overstep the bounds of cold damage." They courageously summed up new experiences, established new theories, and contrived new treatments, until ultimately the achievements of their reasoning on the hot-natured diseases of Chinese medicine led to the cutting of historical ties and the creation of the warm disease system.

During the Qīng Dynasty, several medical experts contributed to the development of the warm disease system. Of these, the achievements of Yè Tiān Shì were the most outstanding. Of those acknowledged through the history of warm disease development, Yè Tiān Shì is considered among the most prominent influences on its being established as a complete system. His oral instructions were organized by his students into a book called the *Treatise on Warm Heat*, one of the most important texts on warm disease logic. In this book, he precisely explains the laws of warm disease outbreak and development, and specifies the defense-*qì*-construction-blood warm disease pattern identification and treatment determination system. This was a major step in the development of warm disease diagnostic methods. He also developed the basic treatment methods. Even today these ideas remain central to the research of warm disease logic. They are an important clinical guideline for pattern identification and treatment determination of warm diseases.

After Yè Tiān Shì, the famous medical expert Wú Jú Tōng wrote a book called the *Detailed Analysis of Warm Diseases* that presented a systematic discussion of warm disease pattern identification and treatment determination. Wú Jú Tōng based this book on Yè Tiān Shì's defense-*qì*-construction-blood theory, supplemented it with a triple burner diagnostic theory, and coordinated both theories. He also summarized the formulas for warm disease treatments into a single complete set, and in so doing constituted the complete system of warm diseases pattern identification and treatment determination.

The medical expert Xuē Shēng Bái wrote a book called *Damp-Heat Disease Chapters* (*Shī Rè Bìng Piān* 濕熱病篇), which advanced and enriched the content of the warm disease system by focusing on the causes and pathomechanisms, pattern identification, and treatment determination of damp-heat disease. Another medical expert, Wáng Mèng Yīng, wrote *Warm Heat Latitudes and Longitudes* (*Wēn Rè Jīng Wěi* 溫熱經緯), which uses the *Classic of Internal Medicine* and *Treatise on Cold Damage* ideas as "latitudes" and *Treatise on Warm Heat* and *Damp-Heat Disease Chapters* as "longitudes." It is a preliminary summary of warm disease theory and experience, and as such contributes towards the development of warm disease as an integrated structure.

CHAPTER 2

WARM DISEASE CONCEPTS

Warm diseases are a category of externally contracted disease caused by warm heat pathogens and marked by signs of heat. The heat in such diseases tends to be strong heat that can easily transform into dryness and damage the *yīn*. Although they result from many different causative factors, occur in different seasons, and during their outbreak and development have many different clinical manifestations, these diseases are always marked by characteristics of warm heat and are therefore called warm diseases.

I. CHARACTERISTICS OF WARM DISEASES

A. WARM DISEASES ARE CAUSED BY EXTERNALLY CONTRACTED WARM HEAT PATHOGENS

Warm diseases are different not only from externally contracted wind-cold but also from internal damage miscellaneous diseases. This is because they are caused mainly by externally contracted warm heat pathogens. Ancient medical experts usually based their perspective about diseases caused by pathogenic warmth on the theory that "externally contracted [diseases] result only from the six [environmental] excesses." They considered that the six environmental excesses transformed into heat and attacked the human body. On the basis of his clinical observations and research, Wú Yòu Kě of the Míng Dynasty determined that warm diseases were caused by a peculiar disease-causing substance of the natural world. Hence, well before the birth of modern pathogenic-microorganism theory, he imaginatively put forward the pestilential *qì* theory of disease origin.

B. WARM DISEASES ARE INFECTIOUS, EPIDEMIC, SEASONAL, AND GEOGRAPHIC

Warm diseases usually possess varying degrees of infectiousness and can be transmitted from person to person via several different entry routes such as the mouth and nose. As Wú Yòu Kě said, "Attack of pathogenic *qì* can be from the heavens or can be from infection." "From the heavens" refers to [indirect] transmission by way of the air; "infection" refers to direct contact. Under certain conditions, warm diseases cause epidemics of varying degree amongst the masses. In ancient times epidemics were called "seasonal movements" or "heavenly currents." As Wáng Shū Hé said:

> *When unseasonable pathogenic qì appears and illnesses manifest with similar symptoms, in old and young alike, this is called seasonal movement of qì. . . .*
>
> *In extreme conditions diseases caused by heavenly movement can spread all over the world; in less extreme conditions they can occur at only one place; in moderate conditions they can occur at only one village, and in mild conditions they can occur at only one household.*

Based on the fact that their incidences follow an obviously seasonal pattern, warm diseases are divided into warm diseases of the four seasons. In regard to the governing *qì* of the four seasons, Chinese medical theory holds that the continuous changes in prevailing climatic conditions engender different pathogens in each season, and that this is why the incidence of warm disease follows an obviously seasonal pattern. In spring for instance, the prevailing weather is warm and windy so diseases are usually caused by wind-heat. In summer, the prevailing weather is hot and very wet so diseases are usually caused by summerheat damp. Some warm diseases also occur at definite geographical locations. Diseases caused by damp-heat, for instance, are usually found in subtropical regions, such as those in southern China.

C. THEIR DEVELOPMENTAL TRANSFORMATIONS HAVE CERTAIN STANDARD RHYTHMS

During warm disease development, the main pathological transformations occur because pathogenic *qì* affects the body's defense-*qì*-construction-blood and triple burner causing loss of regulated functionings and damage to the physical substance of their associated viscera and bowels. Warm diseases that manifest at the exterior usually transmit from the defense aspect, internally, to the *qì* aspect, or even more deeply to the construction-blood aspect. Diseases that manifest at the *qì* aspect can also transmit internally to the construction-blood aspect. Diseases that manifest at the construction aspect can either transmit deeply into the blood aspect or outwardly to the *qì* aspect.

Moreover, according to the theory of transmission through the triple burner, during their initial stage, diseases usually invade the lung defense upper burner. Following this they usually transmit directly into *yáng* brightness or counter-transmit indirectly into the pericardium; then during their final stage they usually damage liver and kidney *yīn*. These are the standard rhythms of the developmental transformations of warm diseases. It should however be recognized that in clinical practice, because of differences in the natures of pathogenic attacks, the physical strength of individual patients, and the appropriateness of prescribed treatments, a specific warm disease will not necessarily follow this rhythm.

D. THEIR CLINICAL EXPRESSIONS HAVE SPECIAL CHARACTERISTICS

The onset of warm diseases is usually acute and fierce; their developments are usually rapid, and their changes are usually frequent. Not only are they marked by fever, but in most cases by exuberant fever with accompanying hot symptoms such as vexation and thirst, red tongue and yellow moss. Moreover, during their courses, the warm pathogen can easily transform into dryness and damage the *yīn*, or fall inward and generate changes that reflect in symptoms such as rashes, vomiting of blood and/or nosebleeds, semi-loss of consciousness, convulsions, and syncope.

II. THE AREA AND CLASSIFICATION OF WARM DISEASES

All externally contracted diseases, except for acute hot diseases caused by external wind-cold, can be classified as warm diseases. The warm diseases discussed in this text include wind warmth, spring warmth, summerheat warmth, damp warmth, autumn dryness, latent summerheat, winter warmth, and warm toxicity. These diseases are usually named after the seasons in which they occur, the governing *qì* of the seasons, or the characteristics of the prevailing climate.

This is illustrated by the following examples. Spring warmth, which occurs during spring, and winter warmth, which occurs during winter, are named according to season. Wind warmth, summerheat warmth, damp warmth, and autumn dryness, although seasonal in their patterns of outbreak, are named according to the governing *qì* of the seasons. Latent summerheat, which occurs during autumn, and warm toxicity, which occurs during winter and spring, are named according to their clinical characteristics. In the former case, the symptoms of summerheat-damp are focused on; the fact that it occurs during autumn and winter is ignored, and the condition is called latent summerheat. In the latter case, the clinical expressions of heat toxins, such as red swelling with hot sensation and pain, are focused on, and the condition is called warm toxicity.

It can be seen from the above that although warm diseases are named according to many different criteria, they are always classified according to their clinical expressions.

Although each of the above-mentioned disease types have their own characteristics, in certain respects they are all very similar. Therefore, to simplify the clinical procedure of pattern identification and treatment determination, they can be identified, according to the nature of their symptoms, as pertaining to one of the two general categories of warm heat and damp-heat. Those that can be classified as warm heat include wind warmth, spring warmth, summerheat warmth, autumn dryness, winter warmth, and warm toxicity. Those that can be classified as damp-heat include damp warmth and latent summerheat. Furthermore, warm diseases can also be divided into new attack and latent pathogen types, according to the different natures of their onset. Those initially starting from the exterior, like wind warmth, autumn dryness, and winter warmth, are newly contracted warm diseases; those starting from the interior, like spring warmth and latent summerheat, are latent pathogen warm diseases.

III. WARM DISEASES AND COLD DAMAGE

Warm diseases and cold damage are two different but closely related concepts. The term cold damage is used in both a broad and narrow sense.

Generally, cold damage is used as a broad term for all kinds of externally contracted hot diseases, including warm diseases. For example, the *Classic of Internal Medicine* says, "Hot diseases are a kind of cold damage." The *Classic on Medical Problems* states even more explicitly, "There are five kinds of cold damage: wind stroke, cold damage, damp warmth, hot diseases, and warm diseases." The cold damage referred to in the "five kinds of cold damage" is the broad-sense cold damage. It includes the narrow-sense cold damage, externally contracted diseases of "wind stroke" and "cold damage," and also the warm-type externally contracted disease of "damp warmth."

The narrow-sense cold damage diseases, included among the five kinds of cold damage, are externally contracted diseases of a wind-cold nature. When used in a broad sense, cold damage refers to both cold and warm diseases, the natures of which are quite different. Thus when warm diseases are classified as broad-sense cold damage, they are seen to be of a lower order; but when warm disease and broad-sense cold damage are compared, as if [they were] two completely different externally contracted diseases types, they are seen to be of the same order.

In clinical practice, warm diseases caused by externally contracted warm heat pathogens, and cold damage caused by externally contracted wind-cold, must be differentiated. This is because although they are both externally contracted, their pulses and treatments are quite different. Warm diseases are caused by attacks of pathogenic warm heat. Initially, the pathogen is in the lung defense, so there are symptoms of external heat such as fever stronger than aversion to cold, thirst, coughing, thin, white tongue moss but red tongue, and floating rapid pulse. These are symptoms that should be treated by using acrid cool exterior-resolving medicinals to course the wind-heat. Cold damage results from externally contracted pathogenic wind-cold. Initially, the cold is trapped at the exterior and the defense *yáng* is confined, so there are external cold symptoms such as aversion to cold stronger than fever, headache, body ache, absence of perspiration, thin white tongue moss, and floating tight pulse. These are symptoms that should be treated using acrid warm exterior-resolving medicinals to dissipate and scatter the wind-cold.

IV. WARM DISEASES AND WARM PESTILENCE

The term "warm disease" refers to externally contracted hot diseases that are of a warm heat nature. The term "warm pestilence" refers to the kind of diseases, among the warm diseases, that are highly contagious and epidemic in nature. These two concepts are different but closely related. Due to their different environments, clinically observable results, and interpretations, the medical experts of ancient times had conflicting views about the relationship between these two concepts. According to one school of thought, warm pestilence was merely a different term for warm disease. In the thinking of this school, since warm diseases are contagious they can also be called warm pestilence. Thus although different in name, these two terms actually refer to the same illness. For example, Wú Yòu Kě said:

> *Hot diseases are the same as warm diseases, but are also called warm pestilence because they go from door to door, recruiting everyone, like the forced-labor campaign from which no one is immune.*

According to another school of thought, warm pestilence is different from warm disease. The distinction, as expounded in this theory, depends on whether or not the diseases are contagious—contagious diseases are called warm pestilence, non-contagious diseases are called warm diseases. As Lù Jiǔ Zhī (陸九芝) said:

> *Warmth refers to warm disease; heat refers to hot disease. There is only one way to differentiate these two types of disease from warm pestilence—by determining whether or not they are contagious.*

In both schools of thought, warm pestilence is considered a class of contagious disease. The only difference of opinion is whether or not warm diseases are different from warm pestilence diseases, or in other words on whether or not warm diseases are contagious. From the modern viewpoint, since these two opinions were formed under certain historical restrictions, they are both rather too narrow. As mentioned before, since warm diseases include various acute contagious diseases and certain acute infectious diseases, they are usually all contagious to varying degrees. There are however obvious distinctions between contagious and epidemic warm diseases. It is therefore just as inappropriate to regard all warm diseases as strongly contagious, confusing them with the concept of warm pestilence diseases, as it is impractical to use contagiousness or non-contagiousness as a basis for comparing warm diseases with warm pestilence diseases. Nonetheless, it was a positive step in the prevention and treatments of these diseases to refer to those that are strongly contagious and epidemic as warm pestilence diseases.

By establishing a clear concept by which the different contagious and epidemic conditions of warm disease could be identified and distinguished from general warm diseases, the importance of preventative treatment was highlighted, and effective preventative measures were introduced to control their spread. The main reason that warm pestilence diseases were not considered an independent class of disease was that their pattern identifications and treatment determinations were too similar to those of the four seasons warm diseases. There have never been any separate discussions in Chinese medical literature on this topic.

CHAPTER 3

WARM DISEASE: DISEASE CAUSES AND DISEASE OUTBREAK

I. DISEASE CAUSES

The principal pathogenic factor to which a warm disease can be attributed is externally contracted pathogenic warm heat (this is abbreviated to pathogenic warmth). Pathogenic warmth refers to a class of external pathogenic *qì* with a warm, hot nature—pathogens such as wind-heat, summerheat-heat, damp-heat, and dry-heat. Characteristically, besides having a warm nature, such pathogens are also transmitted via external contraction and generate diseases very quickly.

The theory of warm disease causes is a summary of the theories of warm disease causative factors, based not only on the clinical characteristics of the warm diseases of the four seasons, but also on the climatic changes that occur during the seasons of their outbreaks. Over long periods of clinical practice, the medical experts of ancient times concluded that the incidence of warm disease outbreak occurs in a characteristic rhythm. They also realized that this rhythm is different from any rhythm associated with the incidence of internal damage miscellaneous disease outbreak (i.e., general diseases such as internal diseases, pediatric diseases, and gynecological diseases), and recognized that the reason for this is that warm diseases are caused by external pathogens. Furthermore, as the technological limitations of ancient times prevented the investigation of pathogenic microorganisms, since all knowledge of external pathogenic *qì* was based on clinical observation and practical experience, the obvious climatic changes were regarded as the main pathogens in nature. Hence the saying, "External contractions do not exceed the six excesses; diseases should be classified according to the four *qì*."

From the modern viewpoint, warm diseases include various acute infectious and contagious diseases, and their outbreaks result from infections by pathogenic microorganisms. Although natural factors like climatic changes influence the reproduction of pathogenic microorganisms and the resistance of the body, they are not the direct causes of warm diseases. According to this understanding, the climatic changes of the four seasons are only one of the factors contributing to the outbreak of warm diseases. Traditionally however, the "six pathogens" were regarded as the main cause of warm diseases and were also used in forming the complete system of seeking disease causes from patterns identified and determining treatments according to causes, a system which even today is still used as the guidelines to clinical practice. Therefore, at present, rather than being construed as simply the physical pathogens in nature, the "six pathogens" must instead be viewed as broad categories that include pathogenic microorganisms. It was only the limited scientific level that prevented this from being clearly recognized in ancient times.

Actually, the significance of warm disease cause theory is not limited to explaining the reasons for the outbreak of warm diseases. It is also more importantly used as a clinical guideline for seeking disease causes from patterns identified and determining treatments according to causes. Besides having obvious seasonal natures, each of the pathogens of the four seasons is associated with specific symptom expressions and corresponding treatment methods. Therefore, in clinical situations one only has to master the characteristic disease-causing features of each pathogen, by analyzing the differing symptom expressions, to accurately distinguish warm disease pathogen types, adopt effective treatment methods, and perform appropriate treatments. This is the gist of seeking disease causes from patterns identified, and determining treatments according to causes. The characteristics of the various warm heat disease pathogens are discussed below.

A. WIND-HEAT PATHOGENS

Diseases caused by wind-heat pathogens usually occur during spring and winter. During spring, *yáng qì* upbears and weather conditions are warm so it is easy for wind-heat to attack the human body. If warm diseases caused by wind-heat attacking the human body appear during spring they are called wind warmth diseases. If unseasonable weather patterns occur during winter so that the weather, which is normally cold, becomes unseasonably hot, and warm heat pathogens take form, the resulting diseases are called winter warmth. Both these diseases require similar treatments.

The wind-heat pathogen is characteristically upbearing and dissipating. When it invades the human body it first attacks the lung system, including the skin, body hair, and external muscles. It can also easily disperse [i.e., loosen] the striae. So, initially, diseases caused by wind-heat pathogens are usually located in the upper burner lung defense. Clinical manifestations of external heat such as fever, slight aversion to wind or cold, mild sweating, coughing, thirst, thin, white tongue moss, red tongue, and floating rapid pulse can therefore be seen. As Yè Tiān Shì said, "Warm pathogens invade above, attacking the lungs first." This summarizes the characteristics of wind warmth disease occurrence.

Another characteristic of diseases caused by wind-heat pathogens is that their onsets and developments are very rapid. Moreover, during their courses, their pathomechanism can easily counterflow into the pericardium. But if their courses run smoothly there are no such difficulties. These pathogens also disappear very quickly, so their pathological processes are short-lived.

B. SUMMERHEAT-HEAT PATHOGENS

When warm diseases occur during summer, they are usually caused by summerheat-heat pathogens. Also, diseases caused by summerheat-heat pathogens have a very obvious seasonal nature. As the *Classic of Internal Medicine* says, "Warm diseases seen before the summer solstice are caused by warmth; warm diseases seen after the summer solstice are caused by summerheat."

This clearly identifies the seasonal limitations of warmth and summerheat. Warm diseases during summer, caused by attacks of summerheat-heat pathogens, are called summerheat warmth.

Summerheat-heat pathogens are extremely hot, so when they invade the human body, the onset and development of disease is usually very rapid. During most such diseases, pathogens enter directly into the *qì* aspect. Defense aspect symptoms are conspicuously absent. Initially there are *yáng* brightness, *qì* aspect symptoms such as vigorous fever, great sweating, thirst, and surging rapid pulses, or in severe cases when summerheat-heat enters directly into the pericardium and liver channels, there are serious symptoms such as clouding reversal.

Summerheat-heat pathogens can easily damage the *qì* and consume the liquid. Therefore, symptoms of summerheat damage to the liquid *qì* are quite commonly seen, and in severe cases serious patterns such as imminent desertion of liquid *qì* can occur.

The weather during summer is very hot. Heat bears down from the heavens, but at the same time damp steams upward from the earth. It is therefore not only heat that is very strong but also dampness. For this reason summerheat-heat pathogens can easily harbor dampness and manifest as patterns of summerheat warmth with dampness. Moreover, since people like drinking cold drinks and sleeping in cool breezes during summer, diseases caused by summerheat-heat pathogens can easily be obstructed by cold dampness, so patterns of summerheat accompanied by cold dampness are also seen quite commonly.

C. DAMP-HEAT PATHOGENS

Damp-heat pathogens exist in all four seasons, but become stronger in long summer. Since the weather between summer and autumn is very hot and very rainy, dampness and heat steam together, and damp-heat diseases are readily seen. Warm diseases that can be attributed to attacks by summerheat-damp pathogens are called damp warmth, while warm diseases that harbor accompanying symptoms of dampness are called wind warmth harboring damp or summerheat warmth harboring damp.

The characteristics of diseases caused by damp-heat pathogens are clearly different from those of diseases caused by other warm heat pathogens. Their main expressions are as follows:

Being a *yīn* pathogen, dampness transforms into heat more slowly than other warm pathogens. Therefore, during the early stages of a damp warmth disease the heat signs are not very strong. There are expressions of unsurfaced fever, slimy white tongue moss, and lack of thirst.

Dampness is turbid by nature. After invading the human body, it lodges and does not transform easily. Unlike diseases caused by cold pathogens, which disappear when sweating is induced, or hot pathogens, which disappear when heat has been cleared, diseases caused by damp pathogens are usually protracted and intractable. Moreover, remissions occur quite commonly, even after apparent recovery.

Damp pathogens can easily damage the spleen and stomach. Both these organs are housed in the middle burner and their main function is to transform water and food. Damp-heat pathogens invade from the exterior, and after entering the body can easily obstruct the spleen and stomach. Therefore, in damp warmth diseases, the core of disease transformation is usually concentrated at the middle burner in the spleen and stomach. Symptoms such as stomach duct dilations, abdominal distention, nausea, and diarrhea occur.

Dampness has a heavy, slimy nature and is consequently easily able to block the clear *yáng* and obstruct the *qì* dynamic. Therefore, during the course of a damp warm disease, damp-heat tends to linger in the *qì* aspect for relatively long periods. By clouding the clear *yáng* and obstructing the *qì* dynamic, it creates symptoms such as feelings of distention and heaviness in the head, yellow complexion, lassitude of the spirit, stomach duct dilations, abdominal distention, and scant urine. When obstructions are prolonged they can damage the *yáng qì*. This is referred to as dampness winning; *yáng* weakening.

D. DRY-HEAT PATHOGENS

When warm diseases occur during autumn, they are usually caused by dry-heat pathogens—pathogens that form when the natural conditions of autumn ensure that the weather remains consistently sunny and dry. The main characteristic of a dry disease is that it easily consumes fluids. Therefore, at the initial stage of a warm dry disease, besides the normal symptoms of external contraction seen in all warm diseases, there will always be accompanying symptoms of liquid damage such as dry mouth, nose, and throat. Also, since dry-heat pathogens usually attack above, via the mouth and nose, the core of pathological change is normally centered in the lung channel.

Apart from the theory that warm diseases are caused by the warm heat pathogens of the four seasons, there is also a theory that they are caused by pestilential *qì*. This theory was advanced by Wú Yòu Kě, a Míng Dynasty medical expert, who explained that warm diseases can be transferred by indirect or direct contact. These are the two distinguishing features of warm disease epidemics. Based on these two characteristics, he posited the concept of pestilential *qì* as a disease cause. In the opinion of Wú Yòu Kě, scourge epidemics are not caused by the six externally contracted *qì* of wind, cold, summerheat, dampness, dryness, and heat, but by another peculiar disease-causing substance of the natural world. When they occur, such diseases are very strong, very severe, and very contagious. He therefore postulated the concept of pestilential *qì*.

This broke away from the idea that "all diseases are caused by the six externally contracted pathogens." Since it was advanced before the discovery of pathogenic microorganisms, this theory was an important development. It was also a major step in the evolution of warm disease pathomechanics. But due to the technological limitations at that time in history, this understanding was based solely on the analysis of sensory inputs, and so was a very limited perspective. Because of its shortcomings, particularly in the area of seeking disease causes from patterns identified and determining treatments according to causes, it was never developed as a separate system. The true significance of the pestilential *qì* theory is therefore limited to its indicating that scourge epidemics have different (epidemic) characteristics than normal warm diseases.

In addition, warm-disease disease causes also contain the concept of warm toxins. Warm toxins, which are also called warm heat toxin pathogens, are pathogens that cause warm diseases with certain special, unique characteristics. Their conceptualization grew from a summary of clinical experience. There are some diseases that besides having the normal clinical manifestations of warm disease also have characteristic signs of local redness, heat, swelling, and pain or ulcerations. These characteristics make them easy to differentiate from normal warm diseases. Because of this, the medical experts in ancient times contrived the concept of warm toxicity. But it can be seen from their nature that warm toxins are actually various types of warm heat pathogens.

II. DISEASE OUTBREAK

A. FACTORS INFLUENCING THE OUTBREAK OF DISEASE

The theory on factors that influence the outbreak of warm disease is based on the *Classic of Internal Medicine* idea that, "When right *qì* is stored internally, pathogenic *qì* cannot attack." This explains that warm diseases occur not only because of external pathogens, but also and more importantly because of the state of the human body's internal functioning (i.e., the strength or weakness of the right *qì*). Warm diseases are a class of externally contracted diseases, but although external contraction is an important causal factor, whether or not warm diseases occur depends on whether or not the external pathogens are able to invade the human body, and, should the external pathogens successfully invade, on the strength or weakness of the right *qì*, and on the struggle between the forces of pathogenic and right *qì*. This means that warm disease pathogens can only invade the human body when the right *qì* is insufficient, the resistance is weak, or the attacking external pathogens are powerful enough to overcome the resisting function of the right *qì*. These are the circumstances under which warm diseases can occur. As the *Miraculous Pivot* states in the *Treatise on the Primary Occurrence of Diseases*:

> *When wind, rain, cold, and heat are normal they cannot damage the human body. But when wind, cold, and rain grow suddenly fierce and people remain healthy, it means that their right qì is strong. When right qì is strong, pathogenic qì is unable to cause damage. Only when pathogens and weaknesses of the human body combine can attacks be successful.*

The occurrence of warm disease depends not only on the internal strength or weakness of the right *qì*, but also on the external environmental factors. The natural weather changes throughout the four seasons affect not only the formation of pathogens but also the resistance of the human body. Different changes result in different warm diseases occurring. For instance, during summer when the weather is hot and dampness is prominent, dampness and heat mix together and damp-heat gets stronger. Moreover, the spleen and stomach functions grow very sluggish, so it becomes easy for damp-heat pathogens to attack. Besides, if the weather becomes unseasonal—if for example it becomes suddenly cold, suddenly hot, cloudless for prolonged periods, or rainy for prolonged periods, this too can contribute to the occurrence of warm disease epidemics.

B. TYPES OF DISEASE OUTBREAKS

Although there are many different factors contributing to the outbreak of warm diseases, based on clinical experience, they can be summarized as two types: new contraction and latent pathogen types. When a warm disease occurs immediately after an attack by an external pathogen it is called a newly contracted disease; when an external pathogen attacks without causing a disease, hides deeply in the body, then reemerges after some time, the resulting warm disease is called a latent disease.

By comparing various warm diseases and analyzing their differences, our predecessors discovered that warm diseases have two possible ways of breaking out—from the exterior and from the interior. The main significance of this discovery was that it enabled theory to explain the different types of warm diseases at their initial outbreak, to identify the severity or mildness of diseases, to predict the direction of their pathological transformations, and to determine appropriate treatment methods. Newly contracted diseases are differentiated from latent attacks according to whether or not symptoms appear immediately after the initial attack of a pathogen. In clinical practice, the principal procedure for differentiating these contrasting types of warm diseases, at their initial stages, is analysis of symptoms. In most cases, newly contracted warm diseases occur at the exterior, with symptoms such as fever, aversion to cold, absence of sweating or slight sweating, headache, coughing, floating rapid pulse, and thin white tongue moss. If the trend of transformation is from the exterior directly into the interior, the condition is usually relatively mild and the disease course relatively short. Initially, the main treatment is to resolve the exterior and outthrust the pathogens.

Most latent warm diseases, on the other hand, emerge from the interior and have main expressions of confined internal heat—symptoms such as scorching heat (i.e., the patient is hot to the touch), vexation, thirst, scant yellow urine, red tongue, and yellow tongue moss. Such conditions are usually relatively more severe than those of newly contracted warm diseases, and the disease course is relatively longer. There are also two possible trends of transformation. Internal heat can outthrust to the exterior, or fall inward and become deeper. Since even at the initial outbreak the disease pathogen is already internal, the main treatment must be to clear and discharge the internal heat. These variations of warm disease outbreak (i.e., new and latent) are influenced by the nature of the pathogen, the strength or weakness of the pathogen, and the resistance of the human body.

Although all latent warm diseases have symptoms of internal heat during their initial stages, there are in fact many different types. Our predecessors therefore used the different clinical manifestations of warm diseases to develop the idea of pathogens being hidden at different locations, of pathogens for instance being hidden in lesser *yīn* or lodging in the *yīn* aspect. Their initial idea was to make the clinical identification and treatment of different symptoms easier.

CHAPTER 4
DIFFERENTIATION OF WARM DISEASE PATTERNS

Warm disease pattern identification is based on the defense-*qì*- construction-blood and triple burner theories. It was developed by the medical experts of ancient times over long periods of medical practice, as they summed up their clinical experiences regarding the trends of pathological change and the corresponding symptom changes during the course of warm diseases. Its particular significance is instructive as a guideline to clinical practice.

I. DEFENSE–*QÌ*–CONSTRUCTION–BLOOD PATTERN IDENTIFICATION

The defense-*qì*-construction-blood system of pattern differentiation was first developed by the medical expert Yè Tiān Shì. By observing warm diseases over a long period of clinical practice he noticed that they had certain trends of development, and also that their pathological changes were expressed mainly as abnormal functionings of or damage to the substances of defense, *qì*, construction, and blood. He found that their symptomatic expressions differed according to the different types of damage that occurred at different locations during different stages of their course, and that their pathological changes and developments were reflected as inter-affecting and inter-transmitting diseases of the defense, *qì*, construction, and blood. He therefore formulated and streamlined the defense-*qì*-construction-blood theory and used it as a guideline for pattern identification and treatment determination.

A. DEFENSE–*QÌ*–CONSTRUCTION–BLOOD PATHOLOGIES AND PATTERNS

1. DEFENSE ASPECT PATTERNS

During their initial stages most warm diseases have clinical expressions of fever, aversion to cold, headache, absence of sweating or scant sweating, coughing, thirst, thin, white tongue moss, somewhat red tongue tip, and floating rapid pulse. But among these symptoms, the most prominent are fever with simultaneous aversion to cold. These are also the key symptoms of a defense aspect pattern.

Defense *qì* spreads over the muscle surface, and its main functions are to warm and nourish the exterior, to regulate sweating by governing the openings and closings of the pores, and to protect the body from external pathogens. During the onset of a warm disease, pathogenic *qì* attacks above, so there are usually lung defense symptoms. Since the lungs correspond with the skin and body hair, it can be seen that the defense [*qì*] must correspond with the lung *qì*—they must connect through. This is why, when the lungs and defense lose harmony, the above symptoms occur. There is fever, because after invading the surface, the pathogens struggle with the defense *qì*.

As the *Classic of Internal Medicine* comments, "When defense *qì* is unable to discharge to the exterior there is fever." There is aversion to cold, because when pathogens obstruct the defense *yáng*, the muscles and skin lose warmth and nourishment, and since warm diseases result from warm pathogens, there is normally stronger fever than aversion to cold. The pathogens are at the exterior so the defense *qì* is confined, the skin and body-hair lose their opening and closing functions, and there is absence of sweating or scant sweating. The head is the meeting place of all *yáng* so when warm pathogens attack the exterior, *yáng* heat upbears, disturbs the clear orifice, and causes headache. The defense *qì* is confined and obstructed so the lung *qì* is unable to connect through and there is coughing. Warm heat pathogens easily damage fluids, so thirst occurs even during the initial stage of the disease, although not normally in a very severe form. The pathogens are at the exterior and are inclined to be hot, so the pulses are floating and rapid. A thin, white tongue moss is associated with the exterior, and a red tongue is a sign of heat so thin, white tongue moss with red tongue tip is characteristic of external heat.

2. *QÌ* ASPECT PATTERNS

This pattern generally develops from a defense aspect pattern. If, rather than resolving, defense aspect pathogens transfer internally, they usually enter the *qì* aspect. Since the focus of the pathology changes, the clinical expressions also change. In most cases, there are symptoms of heat flooding into *yáng* brightness—symptoms such as fever, no aversion to cold but aversion to heat, great sweating, thirst with desire to drink cold drinks, dry yellow tongue moss, and a slippery rapid or surging big pulse. The key symptoms of heat in the *qì* aspect are fever without aversion to cold, thirst, and yellow tongue moss.

Qì is the material basis that supports the life force of the human body. It also acts as the motivating agent for the physiological activities of all organs. When pathogens enter the *qì* aspect, upright and pathogenic *qì* struggle fiercely so fever grows higher. But since pathogens are internal rather than external there is no aversion to cold. *Qì* aspect heat is strong so the tongue moss is yellow. Heat damages the fluids so there is thirst. Internal heat steams outward so there is sweating. And internal heat is strong so there is a slippery rapid or surging big pulse.

When warm pathogens penetrate from the exterior to the interior without entering the construction or blood aspects, the resultant disease patterns are of the *qì* aspect. Certain *qì* aspect patterns will be discussed later in the section on triple burner pattern differentiation.

3. CONSTRUCTION ASPECT PATTERNS

Mostly, construction aspect patterns develop from defense and *qì* aspect patterns, but not always. Occasionally they occur during the initial outbreak of a disease. When pathogenic heat enters the construction, symptoms such as fever that grows stronger at night, thirst but little desire to drink, vexation, insomnia, sometimes delirious speech, and rashes, crimson red tongue, and fine rapid pulse can be seen. Of these, the key ones are fever that grows stronger at night, crimson tongue, vexation, and delirious speech. These are also the symptoms that constitute the characteristic pattern of pathogens entering the construction aspect.

Construction *qì* is derived from the essence of water and food. It circulates in the channels and blood vessels, its main function is to nourish the whole body, and it connects through to the heart *qì*. Therefore, when pathogens enter the construction aspect, the main expressions are of heat damaging the *yīn* construction and disturbing the heart spirit. Heat damages the *yīn* construction so there is fever that grows stronger at night, and a fine rapid pulse. Construction heat upbears so the tongue is crimson and there is thirst but little desire to drink. Heat runs along the blood network vessels, so red rashes can be seen (but not very distinctly). Construction *qì* connects through to the heart, so heat in the construction aspect disturbs the heart spirit and symptoms of disturbed spirit such as vexation, insomnia, and sometimes delirious speech occur.

4. BLOOD ASPECT PATTERNS

Blood aspect patterns usually develop from construction aspect patterns. When heat enters the blood aspect, symptoms of fever, agitation and disquietude, and in severe cases mania, dark crimson tongue, and various combinations of vomiting blood, nose bleeding, blood in the stools, blood in the urine, and/or distinct rashes occur. Of these, the key symptoms are deep crimson tongue and bleeding. Such patterns are objective evidence of heat in the blood aspect.

Blood is derived from construction *qì* and circulates in a continuous, non-stop cycle through the blood vessels. When a pathogen is in the construction aspect, unless it is quickly outthrust to the *qì* aspect, it enters deeply into the blood aspect where it consumes and stirs the blood. The heart governs the blood and stores the spirit, so when warm pathogens attack the blood aspect, there are expressions of strong heat, frenetic movement of blood, and disturbed heart spirit. Heat damages the construction-blood, so the body heat of such patients can scorch the hand, especially at night when this type of fever is normally stronger. Heat disturbs the heart spirit, so there are agitated writhings and in severe cases mania. The deep crimson tongue is a sign of strong blood heat. The pathogenic heat in the blood aspect scorches and damages the blood network vessels, thereby forcing frenetic movement of blood, so vomiting of blood, nose bleeding, blood in the stools, blood in the urine, and/or rashes might also be seen.

B. THE DEPTH AND SHALLOWNESS OF DEFENSE-*QÌ*-CONSTRUCTION-BLOOD PATTERNS AND THEIR TRANSFORMATIONS

The pathological changes and clinical expressions during the course of a defense-*qì*-construction-blood disease reflect the changing locations (deep or shallow) of the attacking warm disease pathogens, the disease condition (severe or mild), and the warm disease transformations. As Yè Tiān Shì said, "Generally, after defense comes *qì*, and after construction comes blood." What this means is that pathogens are not as deep in the defense aspect as in the *qì* aspect, but when they are in the blood aspect, they are deeper than when in the construction aspect.

To elaborate, when pathogens are in the defense aspect, diseases are located most superficially (the patterns are external), the durations are shortest and the conditions are mildest. When pathogens are in the *qì* aspect, diseases are already internal, pathogens grow stronger, and if they get any deeper, the functional activities of the organs tend to be affected. The conditions are more severe than when pathogens are in the defense aspect but the right *qì* is still strong and its struggle with the pathogenic *qì* is fiercer. As soon as the correct treatment is given, the pathogens can usually be resolved at the exterior, and the disease cured. If pathogenic heat enters more deeply into the construction and blood aspects, it not only consumes and damages the blood but also affects the heart spirit. The disease condition is deeper and more severe.

Every step in the course of warm disease development is a transforming of defense, *qì*, construction, and blood patterns from one into another. The occurrence or non-occurrence of these transformations depends on the nature of the warm pathogen, the strength of a patient's resistance, and the appropriateness and timeliness of treatments. As a general rule, there are two ways in which such transformations can develop.

1. They can develop from the exterior to the interior. For example, when a warm disease occurs at the exterior, it usually transfers from the defense aspect to the *qì* aspect and later, more deeply into the construction or blood aspect.

2. They can develop from the interior to the exterior. For example, when a warm disease occurs at the interior, its onset is sometimes marked by construction and blood aspect patterns, and later when it transmits towards the exterior, by *qì* aspect patterns.

When pathogens transmit from the exterior to the interior, the disease condition changes from mild to severe, and conversely when pathogens transmit from the interior to the exterior, the condition changes from severe to mild. During the process of transformation and change, if pathogens in the defense aspect have not yet resolved but there are already accompanying *qì* aspect or construction aspect symptoms, an ailment of both the defense and *qì* or defense and construction is indicated. If pathogens have not yet departed from the *qì* aspect but there are already additional construction or blood aspect symptoms, intensifying of heat at both the *qì* and construction or *qì* and blood is indicated. Clearly, the pattern of defense, *qì*, construction, and blood aspect transformations and changes during the course of a warm disease is not rigidly fixed. It is therefore important to recognize that the key to understanding defense, *qì*, construction, and blood transformations and changes is to understand their patterns. As the medical expert Zhāng Xū Gǔ (章虛谷) said:

> *At the onset of any warm disease, fever and aversion to cold indicate pathogens in the defense aspect. Absence of aversion to cold but aversion to heat and yellow urine indicate that pathogens have already entered the qì aspect. If the pulse is rapid and the tongue is crimson, it indicates that pathogens have entered the construction aspect. If the tongue is crimson and there is agitation and disquietude that prevents sleeping, or delirious speech at night, it indicates that pathogens have entered the blood aspect.*

Although it misses certain indications, this passage describes the type of symptoms that characteristically occur at every stage of a warm disease. It can therefore be used in pattern differentiation as a basis for explaining the transmission of disease.

DEFENSE, QÌ, CONSTRUCTION, AND BLOOD PATTERN IDENTIFICATION			
PATTERN TYPE	PATHOLOGY	SYMPTOMS	KEYS TO PATTERN IDENTIFICATION
DEFENSE			
	Warm pathogens lodge externally and the lung defense loses its diffusing function	Fever, mild aversion to cold, headache, absence of sweating or slight sweating, coughing, thirst, thin white tongue moss, red tongue tip, and floating rapid pulse	Fever, mild aversion to cold, mild thirst, floating rapid pulse, and thin white tongue moss
QÌ			
	Pathogens enter the *qì* aspect and there is steaming of internal heat	Fever, no aversion to cold but aversion to heat, great sweating, thirst with desire to drink cold drinks, dry yellow tongue moss, slippery rapid pulse or big surging pulse	Vigorous heat, no aversion to cold, thirst, and yellow tongue moss
CONSTRUCTION			
	Heat scorches the *yīn* construction and the heart spirit is harassed	Fever grows stronger at night, dry mouth but little desire to drink, vexation, inability to sleep, sometimes delirious speech and indistinct rashes under the skin, crimson tongue, and fine rapid pulse	Fever grows stronger at night, vexation, crimson tongue, and fine rapid pulse
BLOOD			
	Strong heat forces frenetic movement of blood and the heart spirit is harassed and confused	Fever, agitation and disquietude, coma, mania, delirious speech, vomiting of blood, nosebleeds, blood in the urine, blood in the stools, clearly seen rashes, and dark-crimson tongue	Fever and agitated writhing, clearly seen rashes or any symptoms of bleeding, dark-crimson tongue

II. TRIPLE BURNER PATTERN DIFFERENTIATION

The position that triple burner diagnosis now occupies in the Chinese medical system can be largely credited to the work of Wú Jú Tōng, a Qīng Dynasty medical expert. Based on Yè Tiān Shì's experiences regarding the treatment of warm heat diseases, and the ideas derived from his own clinical experience, Dr. Wú devised a system of general laws regarding treatments and symptom patterns during the outbreak and development of warm diseases. He adapted the concept of the triple burner, called his system triple burner pattern identification, and used it not only as a guideline for pattern identification and treatment determination, but also as a means of explaining the process of symptom transformation.

A. TRIPLE BURNER PATHOLOGIES AND PATTERNS

1. UPPER BURNER MANIFESTATIONS

Upper burner manifestations include hand greater *yīn* lung channel and hand reverting *yīn* pericardium channel disease transformations. As Wú Jú Tōng said:

> *In greater yīn diseases the pulses are neither tight nor moderate but moving and rapid at both cùn positions; the forearm skin is hot, and there are also symptoms of headache, mild aversion to wind or cold, fever with sweating, thirst or absence of thirst with coughing, and increasing of heat during the afternoon.*

Warm pathogens enter the human body via the mouth and nose. The nose *qì* connects with the lungs, and the lungs combine with the skin and body hair to govern the defense *qì*. When pathogens invade the lungs, the external defense *qì* becomes confined and obstructed and the lung *qì* loses its ability to diffuse, so the above listed symptoms appear. If pathogens enter internally and pathogenic heat congests the lungs, lung *qì* is unable to diffuse so symptoms of fever with sweating, thirst, coughing, dyspnea, yellow tongue moss, and rapid pulses appear. If lung channel pathogens fail to resolve, enter the pericardium, and close and block the orifice mechanism, there will also be crimson tongue, clouded spirit with delirious speech or coma, short tongue, and limb reversal. As Yè Tiān Shì declared: "When warm pathogens invade above, they first attack the lungs or counter-transfer into the pericardium." This indicates not only that at the beginning of a warm disease the core of disease transformation is in the lungs, but also explains the relationship of disease transformation between the lung and pericardium.

2. MIDDLE BURNER MANIFESTATIONS

Middle burner manifestations include hand and foot *yáng* brightness symptoms and foot greater *yīn* spleen symptoms. *Yáng* brightness and greater *yīn* have an external-internal relationship. Both the spleen and stomach are housed in the middle burner. *Yáng* brightness corresponds with dryness, and greater *yīn* with dampness. When pathogens enter *yáng* brightness there is a tendency for them to transform into dryness. So, in most cases, there are internal, hot, dry, replete patterns. As Wú Jú Tōng comments:

When the complexion and eyes are both red, the voice is rasping, the breathing is rough, the bowels are closed, the urine is scant, the tongue moss is old and yellow or in severe cases black with thorns, there is aversion to heat rather than aversion to cold, and the symptoms intensify at dusk, it indicates that transfer [of the disease] to the middle burner has already occurred—there is a yáng brightness warm disease. If the pulses are floating, surging, and restless, use White Tiger Decoction (Bái Hǔ Tāng); if the pulses are sunken, rapid, and strong, or in severe cases small and full, use Greater Qì-Infusing Decoction (Dà Chéng Qì Tāng).

The patterns described in this passage can be seen when warm pathogens transfer into *yáng* brightness, when heat without form flourishes, or when heat with form binds. When pathogens enter greater *yīn* and transform into dampness, warm dampness symptoms are usually seen. Since the spleen corresponds with dampness and earth, while the stomach is the sea of water and food, these two organs are particularly susceptible to invasions by damp warmth pathogens. The symptoms that can be seen include unsurfaced fevers that do not resolve even after sweating, dilations and oppression in the chest and stomach duct, nausea and desire to vomit, (subjective feelings of) tired heavy body, slimy tongue moss, and slow, short, moderate pulses. These are the main expressions at the initial stage of a damp warm disease. If, after the disease develops, the dampness is confined and transformed into heat, the heat symptoms gradually increase.

3. LOWER BURNER MANIFESTATIONS

Lower burner conditions are expressed mainly as foot lesser *yīn* kidney and foot reverting *yīn* liver symptoms. The kidneys govern storage of *yīn* essence, so when pathogenic heat lingers, without abating, it consumes and detriments the kidney *yīn*. This results in manifestation of symptoms such as fever, red cheeks, heat in the centers of the palms and soles, dry mouth and throat, vacuous pulse, and lassitude of the spirit or vexation and insomnia. The liver is the wind-wood viscus, and so needs to be enriched and nourished by kidney water. If the kidney *yīn* has been so consumed that water fails to moisten wood, the liver loses nourishment and vacuity wind stirs internally. This manifests in symptoms such as trembling hands and feet, or in severe cases convulsions, lassitude of the spirit, limb reversal, palpitations, crimson tongue, scant tongue moss, and weak vacuous pulse. Warm pathogens can easily damage the *yīn* and consume the humor, so when warm diseases enter the lower burner, there are usually symptoms of vacuous liver and kidney *yīn*.

B. THE TRANSFORMATIONS DURING THE VARIOUS STEPS OF A TRIPLE BURNER DISEASE PROCESS

The pathological changes and clinical manifestations of a triple burner disease, as reflected by the viscera and bowels, mark the different steps during the course of a warm disease. Upper burner hand greater *yīn* lung pathological changes usually occur during the initial stage. Middle burner foot *yáng* brightness stomach pathological changes usually occur during the heat abundant stage. Lower burner foot lesser *yīn* kidney and foot reverting *yīn* liver pathological changes usually occur during the final stage. Yet the widely held view that "[Warm diseases] begin in the upper burner and finish in the lower burner" can only be applied to ordinary warm diseases, which break out at the exterior. Since each disease pattern has its own unique nature, it cannot be unequivocally said that every warm disease will begin in the hand greater *yīn* lung channel. In damp warmth, for example, the initial disease changes occur mainly in the foot greater *yīn* spleen—the confinement of pathogens at the external muscles is only secondary. Again, in summerheat wind and summerheat reversal, foot reverting *yīn* liver and hand reverting *yīn* pericardium symptoms occur at the very beginning of the disease. As Wáng Mèng Yīng said:

> *The study of triple burner warm heat theory does not substantiate that all diseases must begin in the upper burner and slowly progress to the middle burner. If latent qì causes an initial outbreak to occur internally, the disease begins in the lower burner. Since the stomach stores impurities, damp warmth pestilence toxin diseases begin in the middle burner and summerheat pathogens harboring damp also invade the middle burner. Summerheat corresponds with fire, and the heart is the fire viscus. Since both have the same qì, summerheat pathogens can easily attack the heart. Even though it begins in the upper burner, this type of disease is not limited to the hand greater yīn channel.*

Therefore during the various steps of a triple burner disease process, the clinical manifestations must be examined and differentiated in each individual disease.

The transformations that occur during a triple burner disease are reflected by the organs. They generally begin in the upper burner hand greater *yīn* lungs, and transfer to the middle burner. This is called direct transference. Transference from the lungs to the pericardium is called counter-transference. If a middle burner disease has failed to heal, it usually transfers to the lower burner (liver and kidneys). As Wú Jú Tōng said:

> *Warm diseases enter the human body via the mouth and nose. [With] the nose qì [they] connect through to the lungs, [with] the mouth qì [they] connect through to the stomach, and when lung diseases counter-transfer, they flow into the pericardium. If left untreated, upper burner diseases can transfer to the middle burner [stomach and spleen], and middle burner diseases, to the lower burner [liver and kidney]. They begin in the upper burner and finish in the lower burner.*

Although commonly seen, the transformations described in this passage do not occur in a rigid, fixed manner. During the process of transformation, middle burner patterns sometimes appear before upper burner patterns have finished, and lower burner patterns, before middle burner patterns have finished.

The aim of pattern identification is to understand the disease so as to ensure that it is correctly treated. In most cases:

> *When pathogens are in the defense, the treatment is to promote sweating. When pathogens are in the qì, the treatment is to clear the qì. When pathogens are in the construction, the treatment is to transfer the heat through to the qì. And when pathogens are in the blood, the consuming and stirring of blood must be addressed so the treatment must be to urgently cool and dissipate the blood.*

also:

> *Treatments [for the] upper burner [must be] mist-like [i.e., upbearing medicinals must be used]; treatments [for the] middle burner [must be] balance-like [i.e., harmonizing medicinals must be used]; treatments [for the] lower burner [must be] authority-like [i.e., downbearing medicinals must be used].*

The concrete treatment methods will be discussed later, in the chapter "Warm Disease Treatments."

The chart summaries on the following page enable the significance of defense-*qì*-construction-blood and triple burner pattern differentiation to be understood. They analyze pathological changes, clearly identify the locations at which pathological changes occur, describe the severity or non-severity of disease dynamics, explain the transformations of disease conditions, and summarize pattern types to enable appropriate selection of treatment methods. When the two charts are compared there are many similarities, but a few differences. Hand greater *yīn* lung defense pathologies, for instance, are similar to pathologies caused by pathogens lodging in the defense aspect, and heat pathogens congested in the lungs, without external patterns, are similar to pathologies caused by pathogens entering the *qì* aspect. But although they are able to be compared to construction aspect patterns, pathologies caused by heat pathogens entering the pericardium do not have the same pathological changes or symptom expressions. In the case of heat congested in the lungs, phlegm-heat is closed internally; in the case of heat entering the pericardium, the *yīn* construction is damaged by heat.

Again, although pathological changes of the middle burner, foot *yáng* brightness stomach, and foot greater *yīn* spleen are able to be compared to *qì* aspect patterns, pathogens in the *qì* aspect are not necessarily expressed as middle burner pathologies. When pathogens are not external but have not entered the construction or blood aspects, they are in the *qì* aspect. Lower burner liver and kidney pathological changes and blood aspect pathological changes are somewhat different. In lower burner liver and kidney pathological changes, the liver and kidney *yīn* have been damaged by heat and there is a vacuity pattern, whereas in blood aspect pathologies, heat forces surging of blood so there is a repletion pattern. From this it can be seen that although a defense-*qì*-construction-blood diagnosis and a triple burner diagnosis have many similarities, they also have a few differences. When applied in clinical practice, they must be inventively combined, so that warm disease pattern identification and treatment determination can be viewed from an all-round perspective.

TRIPLE BURNER PATTERN IDENTIFICATION

PATTERN TYPE	PATHOLOGY	SYMPTOMS	KEYS TO PATTERN IDENTIFICATION
UPPER HEATER			
Hand greater *yīn* lung	Pathogens attack the lung defense and the lung *qì* loses its diffusing function	Fever, mild aversion to wind, headache, thirst, coughing, floating rapid pulse, and thin white tongue moss	Fever, aversion to cold, coughing, thirst, and floating pulse
	Heat pathogens congest in the lung and the lung *qì* is closed and confined	Fever, sweating, thirst, coughing, dyspnea, yellow tongue moss, and rapid pulse	Fever, coughing, dyspnea, yellow tongue moss, and thirst
Hand reverting *yīn* pericardium	Pathogens fall into the pericardium and the heart orifices are obstructed and closed	Crimson tongue, clouded spirit, and delirious speech, or coma with inability to speak, sluggish tongue, and limb reversal	Clouded spirit and delirious speech
MIDDLE HEATER			
Hand *yáng* brightness stomach	Stomach channel heat is exuberant and steaming occurs at the exterior	Fever, no aversion to cold but aversion to heat, very red complexion and eyes, sweating, thirst, rough breathing, dry yellow tongue moss, and floating surging pulse	Vigorous heat, great sweating, strong thirst, dry yellow tongue moss, and floating surging pulse
Hand *yáng* brightness large intestine	Intestinal tract heat binds and bowel *qì* fails to throughclear	Intensifying of fever after dusk, constipation, scant urine, rasping voice, yellow-black very dry tongue moss, and sunken strong pulse	Intensifying of fever after dusk, constipation, yellow-black very dry tongue moss, and sunken strong pulse
Foot greater *yīn* spleen	Damp-heat encumbers the spleen and the *qì* dynamic is confined and obstructed	Unsurfaced fevers that do not resolve even after sweating, dilations and oppression in the chest and stomach duct, nausea, (subjective feelings of) tired heavy body, slimy tongue moss, and soggy moderate pulse	Unsurfaced fevers, dilations and oppression in the chest and stomach duct, and soggy moderate pulse
LOWER HEATER			
Foot lesser *yīn* kidney	Heat pathogens endure and lodge and kidney *yīn* is consumed and damaged	Fever, red cheeks, heat in the centers of the palms and soles, dry mouth and throat, lassitude of the spirit, and vacuous pulse	Heat in the centers of the palms and soles, dry mouth and throat, lassitude of the spirit, and vacuous pulse
Foot reverting *yīn* liver	Water fails to moisturize wood and vacuity wind moves internally	Trembling hands and feet or in severe cases convulsions, lassitude of the spirit, limb reversal, palpitations, crimson tongue, scant tongue moss, and vacuous weak pulse	Trembling hands and feet or in severe cases convulsions, crimson tongue, and vacuous weak pulse

CHAPTER 5
GENERAL METHODS OF DIAGNOSING WARM DISEASES

As a rule, before a disease can be treated it must first be accurately diagnosed. Appropriate treatment usually depends on correct diagnosis. Characteristically, warm diseases have very rapid onsets, frequently changing manifestations, and epidemic natures. Clinically, therefore, it is very important that they be correctly diagnosed at onset, so that effective treatment methods can be adopted as quickly as possible to control their spread.

The main aim of diagnosis is finding the cause in pattern differentiation and determining treatments according to causes, usually from the clinical characteristics of a warm disease. This is done initially by noting their properties and then by analyzing their symptoms (e.g. fever, thirst, sweating, and changes of consciousness). But in order to do this, it is first necessary to distinguish symptoms with special natures from symptoms with general natures. In clinical practice, the observation and analysis of the objective signs that occur during the course of warm diseases—signs such as changes to tongue moss, outbreak of rashes, swollen head and face in massive head scourge, and scarlet eruptions at the skin and muscles in putrefying throat eruptions—can be used not only to identify diseases and patterns but also to differentiate defense-*qì*-construction-blood symptoms from triple burner symptoms. In addition, attention should be paid to the season in which diseases occur.

Although of secondary importance, this property is of undeniable clinical significance. Since all "warm diseases of the four seasons" have a certain seasonal nature, sometimes for conclusive diagnosis to be reached, the season in which a disease occurs and its clinical expressions must be considered together. Wind warmth, for example, usually occurs during spring and winter, spring warmth during spring, and both summerheat warmth and damp warmth during summer and autumn.

Warm diseases are diagnosed solely by the four examinations—inspection, listening and smelling, inquiry, and palpation—the general significance of which are explained in texts on diagnosis. The focus of this chapter is therefore restricted to those areas of examination that are of specific significance in warm disease. These include tongue diagnosis, teeth examination, analysis of rashes, inspection of miliaria alba, and differentiation of warm disease pulses from normal pulses and warm disease symptoms from normal symptoms.

I. TONGUE DIAGNOSIS AND TEETH EXAMINATION

A. TONGUE DIAGNOSIS

Besides having an important place in the four examinations of Chinese medicine, tongue diagnosis has a special significance in the differentiation of warm diseases. It consists of tongue moss examination and tongue body examination—the tongue moss refers to the covering that grows from the tongue-surface, and the tongue body, to the tongue itself. The tongue is the "sprout" and orifice of the heart, the "outer expression" of the spleen, and the site through which many of the body's channels and network vessels circulate. Therefore:

> *Channel-network vessel, viscera-bowel, defense-qì-construction-blood, exterior-interior, yīn-yáng, cold-hot, and replete-vacuous pathologies can all be detected at the tongue. Moreover, since the tongue moss reflects steaming of stomach qì, and the five viscera all depend on stomach qì, the tongue can be used to examine cold, heat, repletion, and vacuity of the five viscera.*

This explains that the internal changes of the human body—such as the repletions and vacuities of the viscera and bowels, the strengths and weaknesses of the *qì* and blood, the sufficiencies and insufficiencies of the fluids, the depth and shallowness of the pathogens, and the cold and hot natures of the conditions—are all reflected in the changes of the tongue. It is therefore not surprising that tongue diagnosis is one of the most commonly used diagnostic tools in warm disease. Clinically, the main elements to examine are the nature and condition, color and luster, dampness and dryness of the tongue moss. Using these to identify the nature of the pathogens, the type of defense-*qì*-construction-blood or triple burner pattern, and the survival or non-survival of the fluids, enables appropriate clinical treatments to be specified.

1. EXAMINING THE TONGUE MOSS

During the course of warm disease, the struggle between pathogenic and right *qì*, the damage to liquid by fever, and the loss of spleen-stomach transforming and transporting functions subject the tongue moss to many types of change. Clinically, therefore, the color and luster, dampness and dryness, thickness and thinness of the moss is examined to determine whether pathogens are in the defense or *qì* aspect, and whether they have a damp or hot nature.

White Tongue Moss

There are two main types of white tongue moss—thin and thick. A thin, white moss normally indicates a defense aspect disease—an external pattern that is generally seen during the initial stages of a warm disease, when the disease condition is milder. A thick, white moss normally indicates a damp pathogen in the *qì* aspect—an internal pattern, usually seen in damp warmth, when damp pathogens are predominant. These types of moss are further subdivided according to whether they are damp or dry.

1. THIN WHITE MOSS WITH INSUFFICIENT FLUID AND SLIGHTLY RED TONGUE TIP: This type of tongue denotes an external warm heat pathogen and is generally seen during the initial stages of a warm disease when the pattern is external and the pathogen is in the defense aspect. White tongue mosses are also seen in wind-cold external patterns, but these can be easily distinguished because when inspected, the moisture and luster of the tongue surface and the tongue color always appear normal.

2. THIN WHITE DRY MOSS WITH RED TONGUE TIP: Tongues like these indicate that unresolved external wind-heat pathogens have damaged the fluids. They are usually seen in patients with pre-existing *yīn* depletion who are also suffering from externally contracted wind-heat.

3. THICK WHITE STICKY SLIMY MOSS: Clinically, this type of moss generally occurs with vomiting of turbid thick sticky foam, and indicates that dampness is obstructing the *qì* aspect. During a damp warmth disease it usually means that dampness is stronger than heat.

4. THICK WHITE DRY MOSS: This occurs when there is non-transformation of spleen dampness, and already damaged stomach liquid. In short, when *qì* is not transforming humor.

5. THICK WHITE SLIMY MOSS WITH CRIMSON-RED TONGUE: This tongue generally denotes trapped dampness and latent heat, a state which when it occurs, usually does so during *qì* aspect conditions, but on occasions can also do so when heat toxins entering the construction are accompanied by non-transforming damp pathogens. In clinical practice, the accompanying symptoms must therefore be considered.

6. THICK WHITE SLIPPERY SLIMY STICKY POWDER-LIKE MOSS WITH CRIMSON-PURPLE TONGUE: This tongue indicates a confinement block of foul turbid damp-heat, and is generally seen when warm epidemic pathogens are latent in the "membrane source."[1]

7. THICK WHITE SODA-LIKE MOSS: This tongue is normally seen in warm diseases with stagnant food harboring latent and confined foul turbidity in the stomach.

8. GRITTY WHITE MOSS: This tongue moss, which is white, dry, and very hard, like sandpaper, denotes stomach heat. It occurs because pathogenic heat transforms into dryness and enters the stomach so quickly that the tongue moss does not have enough time to turn yellow, and because the fluids have already been scorched.

9. MOLDY WHITE MOSS: This indicates that stomach *qì* is debilitated and vanquished, and therefore that prognosis is poor.

In summary, thin white tongue moss is associated with exterior, and thick white tongue moss with interior; moisture and luster implies that fluids remain undamaged; dryness implies that they have

[1]The membrane source (募原 mù yuán) is: 1. The pleura-diaphragmatic interspace; 2. A space between the exterior and interior where warm disease pathogens lodge.

already been damaged. Thick turbid sticky slime usually indicates accompanying foul turbid damp phlegm. As a rule, the white tongue moss is associated with the exterior, with dampness, with mild conditions, and with favorable prognoses. But the gritty white moss that occurs during internal heat bind, and the moldy white moss that occurs after stomach *qì* has been encumbered and vanquished, are associated with the interior, and with severe conditions. These two types of moss should therefore both be considered special cases.

Yellow Tongue Moss

During the development of a warm disease, the tongue moss usually changes from white to yellow. The yellow color denotes internal heat pathogens, and reflects pathogens in the *qì* aspect. As unresolved external warm disease patterns gradually enter internally, the tongue moss gradually changes from white to yellow. In clinical practice, distinctions between thick and thin, moist and dry types must be made.

1. THIN YELLOW MOSS WITH SUFFICIENT FLUIDS: This denotes initial stage pathogenic heat entering the *qì* aspect—prior to fluid damage.

2. DRY YELLOW TONGUE MOSS: This denotes *qì* aspect exuberant heat, and damage to fluids.

3. YELLOW MOSS CARRYING A SLIGHTLY WHITE COLOR, OR YELLOW-WHITE TONGUE MOSS: This indicates that although pathogenic heat has entered the *qì* aspect, the external pathogen has not yet withdrawn.

4. OLD YELLOW CHARRED DRY MOSS WITH THORNS OR CRACKS: This indicates that pathogenic heat is binding and gathering in the stomach—that there is a *yáng* brightness bowel repletion pattern.

5. THICK YELLOW SLIMY TONGUE MOSS OR TURBID YELLOW MOSS: This denotes internal accruing of damp-heat. Normally, when such a moss is seen in a damp warmth disease, unresolved damp-heat has been lingering in the *qì* aspect for quite some time.

In summary, yellow tongue moss is associated with interior, repletion, and heat. When thin, it indicates that diseases are superficial, and when thick, that they are deep. When moist and lustrous, it indicates that liquid remains undamaged, and when dry, it indicates that it has already been damaged. When thick, charred, and dry, it denotes *yáng* brightness bowel repletion, and when thick, slimy, and turbid, it denotes a heat pathogen harboring damp. A yellow moss carrying a white color indicates that external pathogens have not yet terminated—that both the defense and *qì* aspects are diseased.

Gray Tongue Moss

When a gray tongue moss occurs during a warm disease it usually manifests in one of the following three ways.

1. DRY GRAY MOSS: This usually denotes *yáng* brightness bowel repletion with *yīn* humor damage.

2. STICKY SLIMY GRAY MOSS: This indicates an internal obstruction of damp phlegm and normally occurs when warm diseases harbor accompanying phlegm dampness. Clinically, it is usually accompanied by chest and gastric cavity dilations and oppression, preference for hot drinks, and vomiting of frothy saliva.

3. SLIPPERY MOIST GRAY MOSS: This denotes *yáng* vacuity with cold. Clinically, it is always accompanied by symptoms of cold limbs, fine pulse, or vomiting and diarrhea.

In summary, the gray tongue can be associated with cold, hot, vacuity, repletion, or phlegm dampness pathologies. Clinical differentiations must be based on the moisture or dryness of the tongue and the systemic conditions.

Black Tongue Moss

When this moss appears during the course of a warm disease, it usually develops from a yellow or gray moss, and indicates a critical condition with a poor prognosis.

1. DESICCATED OLD-LOOKING DRY BLACK CHARRED TONGUE MOSS WITH THORNS: This indicates intensely exuberant heat toxins with consumed and damaged *yīn* humor patterns. It is normally seen in *yáng* brightness bowel repletion, when failure to treat below leads to internal binding of pathogenic heat and consumption of *yīn* humor.

2. DRY BLACK DESICCATED OR IN SEVERE CASES CHARRED WITHERED MOSS: When this type of moss occurs it is generally seen during the last stage of warm disease, when heat pathogens enter deeply into the lower burner and consume kidney *yīn*. It is usually thin rather than thick and without thorns, so it differs from the black moss in a *yáng* brightness bowel repletion pattern.

3. Black color and moisture over the entire tongue: This denotes a warm disease accompanied by phlegm dampness. It is generally followed by latent phlegm in the chest and diaphragm and is usually accompanied by fever, chest oppression, and preference for hot drinks, but not by critical symptoms.

4. Dry black moss with pale-white lusterless tongue: This occurs during the final stage of a damp warmth disease when damp-heat transforms into dryness, enters the construction-blood, scorches and damages the *yīn* network vessels, and causes severe precipitation of blood, and *qì* deserting with the blood. Since the changes and developments are very rapid in this disease, the tongue moss does not have time to transform. So, although the tongue moss is still very black, the tongue body is already pale. This must not be confused with exuberant heat damaging the liquid, where the tongue moss is black, charred, and desiccated, and the tongue body is crimson-red.

5. Slippery moist black tongue moss without red tongue body: This denotes *yáng* vacuity with exuberant cold and is generally seen during the final stage of a warm disease when *yīn* is exhausted and *yáng* is deserting—when vacuity cold symptoms can be seen.

In summary, although the black tongue moss can be associated with cold, heat, vacuity, or repletion, during the course of a warm disease it is usually a reflection of exuberant heat and *yīn* damage, and it is rarely a reflection of *yáng* vacuity and exuberant cold. Nevertheless, clinical differentiations must be based on the moisture or dryness of the tongue moss, the degree of redness of the tongue body, and the systemic condition.

2. Examining the Tongue Body

The main procedure in tongue body examination is to inspect the color, luster, and form so as to determine whether warm disease heat has entered the construction-blood. Since the tongue is the "sprout" of the heart and the heart governs the blood, when warm disease pathogens enter the heart construction, consuming and stirring the blood, the tongue body must change. The principal categories of change are as follows.

Red Tongue

This means that the tongue has a slightly darker than normal color and usually indicates gradual penetration of heat pathogens into the construction aspect. When warm disease pathogens enter the defense and *qì* aspects, heat pathogens grow progressively more exuberant, and as they do so the tongue tip grows redder and the surface covering appears increasingly grimy. But when heat enters the construction aspect the whole tongue body turns red and the moss ceases to exist.

1. RED TONGUE TIP WITH THORNS: This denotes heart fire flaring upward and usually precedes the development of a crimson tongue body.

2. RED TONGUE WITH CRACKS OR RED SPOTS ON THE TONGUE: This denotes exuberant heart construction heat toxins.

3. TENDER MIRROR-LIKE TONGUE BODY: When inspected, this tongue looks slightly moist but feels dry. It usually indicates that pathogenic heat has just abated, but that fluids have not yet recovered.

Tongue bodies that are pale-red in color, dry, and dull (less red than normal), usually indicate heart and spleen *qì* and blood insufficiency, damaged stomach liquid, and *qì* not transforming humor. Such tongues are usually seen during the final stage of warm diseases, after abatement of pathogenic heat but before restoration of vacuous *yīn*.

Although there are many different types of red tongues that can manifest during the course of warm diseases, when their natures are analyzed they can all be classified as either repletion or vacuity types. Repletion types indicate heat in the heart construction—the tongue body being a vivid-red color. Vacuity types indicate *qì* and construction insufficiency—the tongue body being a faded pale-red color.

Crimson Tongue

This tongue has a dark-red color and occurs when a tongue with a red color develops into a tongue with a deeper red color. It results from similar pathomechanisms and has similar clinical significance to the red tongue, the only difference between the two being in terms of severity. Usually, when the tongue color changes from red to crimson, it means that heat pathogens have entered more deeply. The principal categories of clinically seen crimson tongues are as follows.

1. VIVID-CRIMSON TONGUE: This indicates heat entering the pericardium.

2. DRY CRIMSON TONGUE: This indicates heat entering the construction-blood, exuberant pathogenic heat, and detrimented construction-*yīn*.

3. CRIMSON TONGUE WITH YELLOW-WHITE MOSS: This indicates that although the pathogen has already entered the construction, it has not as yet terminated in the *qì* aspect.

4. CRIMSON TONGUE WITH STICKY SLIMY SURFACE COVERING OR MOLDY MOSS: This denotes heat in the construction-blood aspect harboring turbid phlegm or foul turbid *qì*.

5. CRIMSON MIRROR-LIKE TONGUE: A mirror-like tongue body (i.e., a tongue body with a dry liquidless surface) is an expression of stomach *yīn* debilitation.

6. FADED DRY WILTED CRIMSON TONGUE: This indicates that the kidney *yīn* has been consumed and exhausted and that the patient's condition is very severe.

In summary, the crimson tongue can be divided into repletion and vacuity types. The vivid-crimson tongue and the dry crimson tongue are both associated with heart-construction exuberant heat, while the crimson mirror-like tongue and the faded dry crimson tongue are both associated with damaged *yīn* fluids. There are also differences between crimson tongues that have moss and crimson tongues that do not have moss. If a crimson tongue is accompanied by a yellow tongue moss it indicates a *qì* aspect pathogen that has not yet exhausted, and if it has a slimy, turbid surface covering or a moldy moss it indicates a pathogen carrying turbid phlegm or foul turbid *qì*.

Purple Tongue

These tongues are darker than crimson tongues and usually develop from crimson tongues. A change of tongue color, from red to purple, may occur when construction-blood heat toxins are extremely strong, but may also occur for other reasons. The principal types are as follows.

1. SCORCHED-PURPLE TONGUE WITH THORNS, VERY DARK LIKE A RED BAY-

BERRY: This denotes extremely exuberant blood aspect heat toxins and it is generally seen when exuberant heat stirs blood, or as a premonition of stirring wind tetanic reversal.

2. DARK-PURPLE DRY TONGUE COLORED LIKE PORK LIVER: This denotes liver and kidney *yīn* exhaustion—a critical condition usually with a poor prognosis.

3. DULL-PURPLE BRUISED TONGUE WITH SLIGHT DAMPNESS WHEN TOUCHED: This indicates internal stasis of blood and is usually accompanied by symptoms of blood stasis-like sharp pain in the chest, rib-sides, or abdomen. It can generally be seen in warm diseases harboring residual damage blood stasis patterns.

It should be noted that there is another purple tongue—a pale-purple, greenish, slippery tongue—which indicates a *yīn* cold pattern. Clinically, this tongue usually accompanies vacuity cold symptoms such as aversion to cold, cold limbs, and faint pulse. It is very different from the purple tongue caused by heat and seen in warm disease.

In summary, the purple tongue can be divided into cold and hot, vacuity and repletion types. The scorched-purple tongue with thorns indicates severe heat and exuberant toxins. The dark-purple dry desiccated tongue indicates that the kidney *yīn* is desiccated and exhausted. The dull-purple bruised slightly damp tongue denotes accompanying blood stasis. The pale-purple greenish slippery tongue usually indicates vacuity cold.

3. EXAMINING THE TONGUE FORM

The tongue form is also a very useful source of clinical information. In very simple terms, its main categories are as follows.

1. STIFF TONGUE BODY, VERY INFLEXIBLE AND HARD TO MOVE: This can usually be seen during the final stage of a warm disease when the *qì* humor is insufficient, the network vessels lose nourishment, and there are expressions of stirring wind.

2. SHORT TONGUE BODY: This indicates harassment by stirring internal wind or internal obstruction by turbid phlegm.

3. ROLLED-UP CONTRACTED TONGUE BODY: This indicates that diseases have entered reverting *yīn* and that the condition is critical.

4. Wilting limp tongue body, either immobilized or partially immobilized, unable to be poked out or pulled in: This denotes exhaustion of liver and kidney *yīn*.

5. Deviated trembling tongue: This usually indicates liver wind convulsions.

6. Swollen tongue body covered with slimy yellow tongue moss: This usually indicates rising of smoldering damp-heat toxins.

B. TEETH EXAMINATION

Teeth examination is a special method only used in warm disease diagnosis. As Yè Tiān Shì comments:

> *In warm diseases, after examining the tongue it is also necessary to examine the teeth. The kidneys extend into the teeth, and the stomach network vessels into the gums. If heat pathogens do not dry the stomach-liquid, they must consume the kidney-humor.*

Since warm diseases can easily consume and damage the stomach liquid, [and thus] rob and sear the kidney humor, the teeth must be examined to determine whether heat pathogens are mild or severe and whether fluids have survived or been destroyed.

1. DRY TEETH

The principal teeth to observe are the two front teeth of the upper palate. When the fluid is insufficient or unable to rise and deploy, these teeth lose nourishment and moisture. By observing them, the difference between mild and severe, shallow and deep pathological changes can be ascertained.

1. Shiny dry teeth that look like stones (the surfaces of the teeth appear dry yet lustrous): This generally indicates that although stomach heat has damaged the liquid, the kidney *yīn* has not yet been consumed so the disease is not very severe. But when seen during the initial stage of a warm disease with aversion to cold and absence of sweating, the indication is that the exterior *qì* is not throughclearing, the defense *yáng* is confined and trapped, and the fluids are unable to deploy freely. In such cases, following effusion of the exterior, the

exterior *qì* courses and throughclears, and the fluids rise and deploy, so the teeth dryness disappears.

2. DRY TEETH THAT LOOK LIKE DEAD BONES (THE SURFACES OF THE TEETH APPEAR DRY BUT NOT LUSTROUS): This indicates that the kidney *yīn* has already been consumed and that the prognosis is poor.

2. BLEEDING BETWEEN THE TEETH

The pathologies that cause this symptom can be divided into vacuity and repletion types. Stomach pathologies are associated with repletion, and kidney pathologies with vacuity.

1. BLEEDING FROM THE SPACE BETWEEN THE TEETH ACCOMPANIED BY SWELLING OF THE GUMS: When bleeding is fresh-red in color and abundant, it indicates violent surging of stomach fire and is associated with repletion.

2. BLEEDING FROM THE SPACE BETWEEN THE TEETH BUT WITHOUT ANY SWELLING OR PAIN IN THE GUMS: When bleeding oozes sluggishly from the spaces between the teeth it indicates flaring of kidney fire and is associated with vacuity.

II. RASH AND MILIARIA ALBA DIAGNOSIS

Rashes and miliaria alba that appear during the course of warm diseases are both characteristically occurring, commonly seen signs. Their form, color, luster, and quantity reflect the depth or shallowness, mildness or severity of pathogens, so their examination yields important information for pattern identification and treatment determination.

A. RASH DIAGNOSIS

The red rashes that appear on the skin during the course of a warm disease can be divided according to their form into macules and papules. Usually, both types occur concurrently. For this reason, many of the ancient books on prescriptions used a combination of the characters for macule and papule as a term for rashes.

Form

The differences between macules and papules as they appear at the skin surface are as follows. Macules can manifest in patches, spots, or blotches of brocade-like stripes, which are neither elevated nor depressed. They cannot be felt under the fingers and cannot be made to disappear when pressure is applied. Papules are like indistinct clouds of scattered small granules, or millet grains under the skin. When palpated, they can be felt.

Formative Factors

In warm diseases, both macules and papules are engendered by the same formative factor—internally confined heat entering the construction-blood. However, the specific pathomechanism is different in each case—in one case it is shallow, and in the other, deep. Macules usually result when wind-heat that has been confined to the lungs scurries internally, permeates the construction aspect, and comes out at the blood network vessels. As Zhāng Xū Gǔ said:

> *When heat is blocked in the construction aspect, macules and papules usually occur. Macules emerge at the muscles and are associated with the stomach; papules emerge at the blood network vessels and are associated with the channels.*

And as Lù Zǐ Xián (陸子賢) said:

> *Macules are [associated with] yáng brightness heat toxins; papules are [associated with] greater yīn wind-heat.*

These passages not only explain that diseases responsible for papules occur at a different location from diseases responsible for macules, that one occurs in the lungs and the other in the stomach, but also that their pathomechanics are different, that one is deep and the other shallow.

Diagnostic Significance

Outthrusting of macules and papules to the exterior indicates that pathogenic *qì* is resolving. Their outbreak, in moderate numbers, is therefore considered a positive sign, whereas their outbreak in prolific numbers is considered a negative one. When warm disease heat enters the construction-blood, if macules and papules outthrust but not very distinctly, it indicates that pathogenic heat is closed internally but starting to resolve, so it is a positive sign. However, if the macules and papules are prolific in number, it means that the pathogens are heavy and the toxins exuberant, so it is a negative sign. To a certain degree, as macules and papules outthrust to the surface they reflect the internal pathological changes of the disease. So in clinical practice their color, luster, form, and distribution can be observed to determine whether warm disease pathogenic *qì* is superficial or deep, mild or severe, and whether the body's *qì* and blood are strong or weak. This information enables prognostic predictions to be made and treatments to be determined.

1. OBSERVING COLOR AND LUSTER

Regardless of whether they are composed of macules or papules, red rashes that are consistently red, vivid, luxuriant, and sleek are normal. A red color that is not too dark indicates that heat toxins are mild and superficial. A rouge-red or cock's comb-red color indicates that heat toxins are exuberant. A black color indicates that heat toxins are extremely severe and that the condition is critical, but not necessarily that the prognosis is poor.

Prognosis depends on the strength or weakness of the right *qì*. If for instance there are black mirror-like macules, besides indicating that heat toxins are deep and severe, these also indicate that *qì* and blood are still strong. If correct treatments are implemented, the patient will recover. A black color that is indistinct but surrounded by a circle of red not only indicates that confined fire is concealed internally but also that *qì* and blood are still surviving. Hence, during treatment, if large doses of heat-clearing outthrusting medicinals are administered, in some cases the rashes change from black to red and the disease can be cured. If black rashes look dull, not only do they indicate fixation and binding of heat toxins, but also that right *qì* has perished. Prognosis therefore is usually poor.

2. OBSERVING FORM

Macules and papules can be lax and floating or tight and restrained. The relationship between these two forms indicates whether the disease condition is severe or mild and whether the prognosis is poor or good. As Yú Shī Yú (余師愚) declared:

Macules and papules, once seen, must be carefully observed to clearly distinguish lax and floating from tight and restrained. It can then be immediately predicted whether the patient will live or die.

In other words, if papules and macules are lax and floating with a sleek look, like splashes under the skin, this indicates that the pathogenic toxins are discharging to the exterior—in short, that it is a serious case with steady improvement, and usually a good prognosis. On the other hand, if the papules and macules are tight and restrained, like a row of stitches or arrow-pierced targets, this indicates that heat toxins are very deep and heavy, binding, and difficult to resolve—in short, that it is a serious case with a poor or unfavorable prognosis.

3. OBSERVING DISTRIBUTION

The distribution of macules and papules, whether clustered or diffuse, reflects the mildness or severity of pathogenic toxins. When macules and papules emerge in regular or irregular clusters or diffuse groups, they indicate that heat toxins are mild and shallow and that prognosis is generally good. But when rashes appear rapidly, in clusters, and then join together into patches, they indicate that heat toxins are very deep and extremely severe, and that prognosis is poor. As Yáng Shì Yíng (楊士瀛) remarked:

When macules and papules are diffuse with a fresh red color, they are usually easy to treat, but when they are like brocade stripes or indistinct pancakes their treatment is difficult.

This [comment] draws attention to the relationship between the distribution of macules and papules (whether clustered or diffused) and the prognosis.

4. CONSIDERING RASHES TOGETHER WITH PULSES AND SYMPTOMS

After macules and papules appear at the surface, the pathological changes, as reflected in the pulses and symptoms, are different than before they appear. Therefore, integrating data on the different types of rashes with findings from the analysis of pulses and symptoms can facilitate pattern identification. Before the outbreak of macules and papules there are usually symptoms of vigorous fever, absence of sweating, and vexation. But if there is also the symptom of serious oppression, or in severe cases deafness, an outbreak of macules is indicated, whereas if accompanying symptoms of chest oppression and coughing occur, an outbreak of papules is indicated. As it says in the *Expanded Treatise on Warm Heat* (*Guǎng Wēn Rè Lùn* 廣溫熱論), "Vexation without thirst, red eyes but white tongue indicates that macules and papules will emerge."

After rashes have clearly emerged, fever normally diminishes and the mind becomes clear. This indicates that the pathogens have already outthrust to the exterior, and is a sign of external resolution and internal harmony. However, if macules emerge but fever fails to diminish, or they emerge indistinctly, or as they emerge they remain hidden under the skin and the mind remains clouded, it indicates that the right *qì* is unable to defeat the pathogenic *qì* and that toxic fire is closed internally. These signs reflect a very severe condition.

The outbreak and transformation of macules and papules have certain standard rhythms, and as a consequence there are certain treatment principles that must be observed. Medical experts of ancient times remarked, "Macules must be [treated by] clearing and transforming, must not be [treated by] outthrusting; papules must be [treated by] outthrusting, must not be [treated by] reinforcing *qì*."

Macules are caused by *yáng* brightness dry-heat forcing its way into the blood aspect, and papules, by greater *yīn* wind-heat running internally into the blood network vessels. Therefore, if a patient is suffering from macules, the treatment must be to clear the stomach and resolve toxins, cool blood and transform macules, and if a patient is suffering from papules, to diffuse the lungs and outpush pathogens, clear construction and outthrust papules.

If papules and macules occur concurrently, the principal treatment must be to transform the macules, and the accompanying treatment must be to outthrust the papules. Cool draining medicinals should not be used too soon after the initial outbreak because they can prevent papules and macules from outthrusting to the exterior by trapping and concealing pathogenic heat. If particularly severe congesting and stagnating of internal repletion prevents papules from outthrusting easily, the mild downward-throughclearing method must be used. Reinforcing upbearing medicinals are contraindicated for both macules and papules because if used erroneously they always cause pathogenic heat to close internally, producing severe symptoms such as syncope, coma, and tetanic reversion.

There is another type of macule, sometimes seen in vacuity cold patterns, which is quite different from the macule seen in warm diseases with repletion fire. In clinical practice, these two types of macule must be carefully differentiated.

B. MILIARIA ALBA DIAGNOSIS

miliaria alba are tiny, unsurfaced, fluid filled, white-colored blisters. They look like sparkling diamonds and usually occur on the neck, chest, and abdomen, although on rare occasions they can also occur on the head, face, and four limbs. As they disperse, scales are usually shed.

Miliaria alba generally take form when damp-heat pathogens linger for prolonged periods in the *qì* aspect, stagnate rather than resolve, confine to the muscles and skin, and steam in a fermentation-like process. They are therefore usually seen in warm diseases with damp-heat natures—damp warmth, summerheat warmth harboring damp, and latent summerheat—and in particular, when instead of being treated with clearing light opening discharging medicinals, warm diseases are erroneously treated with enriching slimy medicinals that promote confinement rather than transformation of damp.

The clinical observation of miliaria alba diseases shows that heat is usually expelled with sweating. Prior to their outbreak, there is confinement of dampness and steaming of heat, so the chest is normally affected by uncomfortable oppression. After their outbreak, the pathogens have already been outpushed to the exterior, so chest oppression partially resolves. Since damp-heat pathogens are sticky and slimy by nature, they are unable to be outthrust at a single action, so not all miliaria alba emerge at the same time. Normally, more appear every time fever recurs and the patient sweats.

The principal significance of miliaria alba diagnosis is that it enables not only the nature of pathogens, but also the strength or weakness of liquid *qì* to be differentiated. Whenever a warm disease is accompanied by an outbreak of miliaria alba, a damp-heat disease is indicated. But to proceed further, and differentiate the relative strengths of the pathogenic and right *qì*, the form and clinical expressions of the blisters must also be considered.

When miliaria alba sparkle like diamonds, have a very full form, and are particularly clear, and when after their outbreak fever diminishes, consciousness clears, and discomfort vanishes, this indicates that the liquid and *qì* are both sufficient, that the right *qì* can defeat the pathogenic *qì*, and that the pathogenic *qì* can outpush to the exterior. These signs are favorable. Conversely, when miliaria alba look like dead bones and have a deflated form, or fever fails to diminish and consciousness remains clouded, it indicates that the liquid and *qì* have both perished, that the right *qì* is unable to defeat the pathogenic *qì*, and that the pathogenic toxins can sink internally. These signs are unfavorable.

Since miliaria alba result from damp-heat being confined in the *qì* aspect and lingering there for prolonged periods, and since the pathogens are internal rather than external, in the *qì* rather than the defense aspect, the ancients have said, "Miliaria must be treated by clearing *qì* rather than by resolving and scattering." Here, "clearing *qì*" means outthrusting heat, transforming damp, diffusing and freeing the *qì* dynamic. If the liquid and *qì* have both perished, *yīn*-nourishing, *qì*-boosting treatments must be administered without delay.

III. DIFFERENTIATION OF PULSES

Pulse-taking is an important part of warm disease diagnosis. But since it is only a single diagnostic method, for the entire picture to be grasped, when applied clinically it must always be considered with the patient's overall condition. Some of the pulses most commonly seen during the courses of warm diseases are discussed below.

A. FLOATING, SURGING, RAPID, AND SLIPPERY PULSES

1. THE FLOATING PULSE

This pulse is associated with the exterior and denotes pathogens in the defense aspect. During the initial stages of a warm disease, when the pathogens are in the defense aspect, the pulse is normally floating and rapid. If the pulse is floating, big, and hollow, there is strong heat and the liquid *qì* is already vacuous. If the pulse is floating and hasty, the heat has been confined internally and has not been given the opportunity to outpush.

2. THE SURGING PULSE

This pulse is floating and big or floating and strong. It is associated with patterns of heat and repletion, and is usually seen when strong heat is affecting the *yáng* brightness *qì* aspect. If the pulse is surging, big, and hollow, there is strong *yáng* brightness heat, and the liquid *qì* has been damaged. If the pulse is surging and big, but felt only at the inch positions, heat has damaged the lung *qì*.

3. THE RAPID PULSE

This pulse is associated with heat patterns and normally occurs in combination with other pulses. If, for example, the rapid pulse occurs in combination with the floating pulse, there are warm pathogens at the exterior. If the pulse is rapid, surging, big, and strong, it denotes strong *qì* aspect heat. If the pulse is racing, it indicates confinement of heat internally. If the pulse is rapid and fine, it usually shows that heat has entered the construction-blood and that the construction *yīn* has been consumed, or that heat has invaded the lower burner and that the true *yīn* has been detrimented. If the pulse is vacuous and rapid, then the pathogens are relatively mild, and the vacuity is relatively severe. Such a pulse indicates vacuous heat internally.

4. THE SLIPPERY PULSE

This pulse indicates strong heat with replete pathogens and plentiful right *qì*. If the pulse is slippery and string-like, it usually denotes phlegm-heat gathering and binding. If the pulse is soggy, slippery, and rapid, it usually indicates steaming together of dampness and heat.

B. SOGGY, MODERATE, STRING-LIKE, AND SUNKEN PULSES

1. THE SOGGY PULSE

This pulse usually indicates damp blockage. If the pulse is soggy and rapid, it denotes damp-heat steaming. If the pulse is soggy, moderate, and small, it indicates lingering of strong pathogenic dampness. If the pulse is soggy and fine without enough strength, there is a chronic disease with vacuity of right *qì* because stomach *qì* has not yet recovered.

2. THE MODERATE PULSE

This pulse usually appears in combination with the soggy pulse and is generally seen in damp warmth when the *qì* dynamic loses its diffusing and freeing function. It can also appear in chronic diseases where the stomach *qì* has not yet recovered but, in such cases, it is without power.

3. THE STRING-LIKE PULSE

When a string-like fine moderate pulse appears at the initial stage of a damp warmth disease, it usually indicates that pathogens are blocked in the *qì* aspect. A string-like rapid pulse denotes heat confined in lesser *yáng*—strong gallbladder heat. If the pulse is string-like and slippery, it usually indicates phlegm-heat. If the pulse is extremely string-like and rapid, it denotes strong heat pathogens causing internal movement of liver wind.

4. THE SUNKEN PULSE

This pulse indicates an internal pattern. Generally, it indicates internal binding of repletion pathogens, but may also occur in vacuous patterns. If the pulse is sunken, replete, and very strong, there is either a *yáng* brightness bowel repletion pattern, or a lower burner blood amassment pattern. If the pulse is sunken and weak, or sunken and without power, it usually denotes that the bowel repletion has not yet been eliminated but that the fluids have already become vacuous. If the pulse is sunken, fine, and rough, it indicates that the true *yīn* has been consumed and damaged.

IV. DIFFERENTIATION OF OTHER COMMONLY SEEN SYMPTOMS

During the course of warm diseases, the pathological changes of the defense, *qì*, construction, and blood, and of the viscera and bowels give rise to numerous different symptoms. However, in many cases such symptoms can result from any one of a number of different formative factors and pathomechanisms, besides which each formative factor and pathomechanism is capable of creating a progression of different symptoms. Therefore it is important that each condition be carefully identified and its terms of analysis specified. In other words, commonly seen symptoms with general natures should be distinguished from commonly seen symptoms with special natures. This allows the characteristics of the formative factors and pathomechanisms of warm diseases to be determined, providing valuable insights, and fostering accurate pattern identification. The following section discusses the differentiation of main symptoms that commonly occur during the course of warm diseases.

A. FEVER

Fever is one of warm disease's most prominent symptoms. It is seen in almost every case, usually as a direct result of contracting warm heat disease pathogens.

Warm disease fever is one of the systemic symptoms that manifests when the human body is affected by heat pathogens. It always occurs whenever pathogenic and right *qì* struggle with each other, so on one level it is an indicator of struggle between right and pathogenic *qì*. But in severe cases it may also consume liquid *qì* and detriment the body, so it is also a pathogen that can cause irreparable damage.

Warm disease fevers can be divided into vacuity and repletion types. As a general rule, during the initial and middle stages of fever, there is a fierce struggle between pathogenic and right *qì*, so *yáng* heat is exuberant and usually associated with repletion. During the final stage, lingering pathogenic heat consumes *yīn* liquid, so heat is usually associated with vacuity. Sometimes, however, *yīn* grows vacuous while *yáng* heat is still intense, so that there is a complex combination of repletion and vacuity. In short, the expressions of fever change in accordance with the changes of the pathomechanism. For the nature of a fever to be correctly ascertained in every case, it must be considered in combination with all other symptoms. The various types of warm disease fevers are discussed below.

1. FEVER WITH AVERSION TO COLD

The simultaneous appearance of fever and aversion to cold is associated with the initial stage of a warm disease and is indicative of pathogens in the defense aspect.

2. ALTERNATING FEVER WITH AVERSION TO COLD

These are associated with confinement of heat in lesser *yáng* and are indicative of gate mechanism inhibitions.

3. VIGOROUS FEVER

These are severe fevers in which aversion to cold has already resolved. There is high fever with aversion to heat. These fevers are associated with the entry of pathogens from the exterior to the interior and reflect an intensifying of the struggle between pathogenic and right *qì*. They indicate vigorous *qì* aspect heat.

4. AFTERNOON TIDAL FEVER

These are fevers that intensify during the afternoons. They are associated with binding of heat in the intestinal bowel and are indicate *yáng* brightness bowel repletion.

5. UNSURFACED FEVER

These occur when lingering heat fails to produce strong signs. They are associated with damp-heat in which dampness is relatively stronger and heat relatively milder, and are indicative of dampness that harbors smoldering heat being confined and steaming in the *qì* aspect.

6. NIGHT FEVER

These are fevers that intensify at night. They are associated with pathogenic heat transferring into the construction, robbing and scorching the construction-*yīn*.

7. NIGHT FEVER THAT ABATES AT DAWN

These are fevers that intensify at night but abate at dawn without sweating. They are associated with lingering residual pathogens concealed in the *qì* aspect.

8. LOW FEVER

These occur during the final stage of warm diseases. They are chronic, non-stop and marked by relatively strong heat in the palms and soles. They indicate liver and kidney *yīn* vacuity with diminishing pathogens and increasing vacuity.

B. NORMAL AND ABNORMAL SWEATING

Sweating is a normal physiological function, but during warm diseases where right and pathogenic *qì* struggle where *yīn* and *yáng* loose balance, its expressions are generally abnormal.

1. ABSENCE OF SWEATING

When seen during the initial stage of a warm disease, absence of sweating indicates that the pathogens are assailing the defense exterior, the defense *qì* is confined, and the interstices are blocked. Consequently, there must be defense aspect symptoms such as fever and aversion to cold. When pathogenic heat enters the construction, there are usually symptoms of heat pathogens consuming and scorching the construction-*yīn* and robbing the fluids. The production of sweat is curbed and there are symptoms such as vexation, agitation, and scorching heat without sweating.

2. INTERMITTENT SWEATING

Fevers associated with intermittent sweating, which reduce with sweating but recur later, usually indicate confinement and steaming of damp-heat pathogens.

3. GREAT SWEATING

Great sweating accompanied by high fever, vexation, and thirst indicates intense heat in the *qì* aspect. This results when heat forces fluids to discharge from the interior to the exterior, and is indicative of a fierce struggle between right and pathogenic *qì*. Sudden great sweating or non-stop dribbling of sweat, accompanied by dry mouth, red tongue, rapid big pulses, and clouded spirit, indicates perishing and desertion of *yīn*. Great sweating with ice-cold limbs, hidden pulse, and pale tongue indicates desertion of *qì* and perishing of *yáng*.

4. SHIVER SWEATING

Shiver sweating is sudden head-to-toe shivering followed by sweating over the entire body. It usually occurs when heat pathogens linger in the *qì* aspect and indicates that right and pathogenic *qì* are locked in a struggle that neither is winning. It is an expression of right *qì* trying to drive pathogenic *qì* outward to the exterior. After shiver sweating, pathogenic *qì* usually follows sweat to the exterior and resolves—fever abates, the body cools, the pulses calm, and there is recovery. But in a minority of patients, sweating fails to occur after the body shivers, or fever fails to abate after shiver sweating, and accompanying symptoms of vexation, agitation, and racing pulses occur. In cases such as these, right *qì* is too weak to eliminate pathogenic *qì*, so heat pathogens fall internally. The condition is severe and there are likely to be numerous relapses. It is therefore essential to provide appropriate treatments so that the imminent relapses can be curtailed.

C. HEAD AND BODY PAINS

Head and body pains, which are also called headaches and body aches, can occur concurrently or in isolation. When headaches and body aches occur in warm diseases, they usually result from pathogenic *qì* entering the superficial muscles, and *yáng qì* being confined by the pathogens. They are generally seen during the initial stages. To understand head and body pains, pay attention to their degree of severity, their location, and their accompanying symptoms.

1. Headaches that occur during the initial stage of a warm disease and are accompanied by symptoms of aversion to cold, fever, and absence of sweating or scant sweating, indicate wind-heat assailing the lung defense.

2. Headaches accompanied by red eyes and sore throats usually indicate wind-heat rising and drying the clear orifice.

3. Stabbing headaches or sharp body aches with aching joints, accompanied by vigorous fever, thirst, and manic agitation, indicate heat toxins at both the exterior and interior, following the channels upward.

4. Sensations of distention at the head and eyes, which feels like a turban wrapped around the skull, generally indicate damp pathogens clouding the clear *yáng*, and are usually seen during the initial stages of damp warmth patterns.

5. Sensations of heaviness with aching and pain of the trunk, but not the limbs, are usually caused by damp pathogens obstructed and stagnant in the muscle exterior.

D. THIRST

Thirst is one of the most commonly seen warm disease symptoms. Being a *yáng* pathogen, warmth easily damages liquid and consumes humor, so during the course of a warm disease, it is normal for the symptom of thirst to occur. However, just as there are different degrees to which the fluids can be consumed and damaged, so there are different degrees of thirst. Generally, when warm disease pathogens are in the defense aspect, thirst is relatively mild, but when pathogenic heat transfers into the *qì* aspect and exuberant heat further damages the liquid, desire to drink gets much more severe. Thirst can also appear in warm diseases when accompanying phlegm-rheum or confined dampness that fails to transform prevents *qì* from distributing liquid.

Sometimes thirst is marked by a desire to drink and sometimes by no desire to drink. Sometimes there is a desire to drink hot drinks and sometimes cold drinks. A desire to drink cold drinks is usually a sign of exuberant *yáng* brightness heat with damaged liquid, whereas thirst with a desire to drink hot drinks or thirst with no desire to drink are indications of either accompanying phlegm-rheum or confined dampness.

When a patient has a dry mouth but is not thirsty, it indicates warm disease pathogenic heat has entered the construction, and that the construction *yīn* has been scorched.

When bitter taste in the mouth accompanies thirst, it usually indicates intense gallbladder fire internally. When loose, unformed stools accompany thirst, it usually indicates *yáng* brightness heat diarrhea.

E. VOMITING

When vomiting occurs during warm disease it is primarily associated with the stomach losing its harmonizing and downbearing functions. The stomach governs intake and normally harmonizes upbearing and downbearing, but if invasions by external pathogens, or damage by food, cause it to lose these functions, the ascending counterflow of stomach *qì* that consequentially follows results in vomiting.

When vomiting occurs in a warm disease, it normally occurs during the initial stage and is accompanied by symptoms such as aversion to cold, headache, and body ache. Usually, it results from external pathogens that lodge at the exterior and invade the stomach, but when it is relatively severe and accompanied by oppression in the chest and slimy tongue moss, it is generally attributable to dampness obstructing the middle burner and turbid *qì* counterflowing upward.

When vomiting of sour vomitus is accompanied by hiccoughing and loss of appetite, or vomiting of undigested food is accompanied by abdominal distention and fullness, there is usually associated loss of the harmonizing and downbearing functions of the stomach caused by retention of stagnant food internally. This is usually seen when warm diseases are accompanied by food stagnation.

Vomiting of clear fluid or copious phlegm, or retching with a bitter taste in the mouth, is associated with retention of damp-heat, and with liver and gallbladder fire counterflowing upward. When one of these occurs, it usually occurs in a damp warmth disease.

When thirst and diarrhea accompany vomiting, and scorching heat occurs at the anal gate, stomach and intestinal heat are indicated.

Frequent vomiting accompanied by high fever, rigidity of the neck, extremely severe headache and sometimes convulsions, is associated with internal movement of liver wind and is normally seen when heat toxins flare upward and counterflow into *yáng* brightness.

Non-stop vomiting in a patient with a thin, weak physique and a mirror-like red tongue is associated with severely damaged stomach *yīn* vacuity [causing] stomach *qì* counterflow, and is usually seen during the final stage of a warm disease.

F. PAIN AND DISTENTION IN THE CHEST AND ABDOMEN

The chest and abdomen are two different areas, so the pathological changes in the diseases that cause pain and distention in the chest occur at different locations from the pathological changes in the diseases that cause pain and distention in the abdomen. Also, pain and distention are two different symptoms; each can appear in isolation or both can occur together. When they occur together, the types of pain and distention that accept pressure are different from the types that refuse pressure. The types that accept pressure are associated with vacuity, whereas the types that refuse pressure are associated with repletion.

Pain and distention in the chest and abdomen are usually associated with a loss of *qì* dynamic function due to damp obstruction, or accumulation and stagnation, or blood stasis. In clinical practice, the underlying cause must be identified.

When chest pain is accompanied by fever and coughing, or coughing of phlegm that is difficult to expectorate, and coughing aggravates chest pain, it indicates that the network vessels are being damaged by lung heat and that lung *qì* is inhibited. If the chest is oppressed and the breathing is shallow or the coughing lacks power, it usually indicates lung *qì* vacuity.

Chest and rib-side pain accompanied by fever and bitter taste in the mouth are associated with confined heat in the liver and gallbladder.

Dilations and oppression in the chest and stomach duct, accompanied by vomiting and thick slimy tongue moss, are usually associated with confinement and stagnation that results from dampness obstructing the *qì* dynamic of the spleen and stomach. If accompanied by belching with a rotten sour odor and aversion to food there is usually accompanying food stagnation.

Alternating abdominal pain and dark-colored diarrhea with slimy yellow tongue moss is usually associated with damp-heat harboring food stagnation, obstructing and stagnating in the intestinal passage.

Very painful, hard fullness in the lateral lower abdomen, accompanied by clouded spirit, delirious speech or manic confusion, black stools, and crimson-purple tongue, usually indicates amassment of blood in the lower burner. However, it can also be seen in women suffering from warm diseases, when heat enters the chamber of the blood.

G. ABNORMAL ELIMINATION OF URINE AND STOOLS

During the course of a warm disease, abnormal elimination is usually associated with loss of control by the intestinal passage over its secreting and conveying functions, loss of control by the bladder over its *qì*-transforming function, or fluid vacuity. Abnormal elimination refers mainly to any abnormal frequency, nature, and/or color of the urine and/or stools.

Slightly yellow urine with chills, fever, and headache indicates the initial stage of a warm disease with heat mainly at the exterior—interior heat is not very severe.

Scant dark yellow urine is usually associated with a repletion heat pattern and is normally seen in a warm disease with intensifying of heat in the *qì* aspect.

Dribbling of urine or in severe cases scant urine followed by anuria usually indicates damp-heat smoldering and binding in the lower burner with a loss of bladder *qì*-transforming function, or desiccated fluids with a damaged source of transformation.

Constipation accompanied by painful abdominal distention that refuses pressure and dry yellow tongue moss with thorns manifests a *yáng* brightness bowel repletion pattern.

Severe constipation, in which stools are only passed once every several days, with accompanying symptoms of dry mouth and red tongue, usually only occurs during the final stages of warm disease, after the liquid has been desiccated and the intestines have dried.

Diarrhea that is hot and malodorous with fever, red tongue, yellow tongue moss, and rapid pulse usually indicates an intestinal heat pattern.

Diarrhea that is completely watery and extremely malodorous and that creates scorching heat at the anus is called heat bind with circumfluence.

Diarrhea that is ochre in color with unsatisfying defecation that creates scorching heat at the anus indicates damp-heat harboring stagnation and obstructing the intestinal passage.

H. ABNORMAL CONSCIOUSNESS

In warm diseases, abnormalities of consciousness are usually associated with the heart spirit. Since the heart governs the mind, the faculty of speech, and the entire body, when disease pathogens invade and interrupt the heart spirit, abnormal consciousness must occur. Abnormal consciousness is usually expressed as vexation and agitation, somnolence, and clouded spirit with delirious speech. Because clouding of the spirit and delirious speech usually occur together, they are habitually referred to as clouded spirit with delirious speech.

The principal characteristic of clouded spirit with delirious speech is abnormal consciousness with divagation and inability to deliberate. When deep loss of consciousness is unaccompanied by delirious speech it is called coma.

When loss of consciousness occurs during warm diseases, it usually occurs in closure patterns and repletion patterns, so the primary imperative is to differentiate heat closures from phlegm coverings. In heat closures resulting from heat pathogens invading the pericardium and causing internal closure of the clear orifice, the subsequent loss of consciousness is very deep. There can be delirious speech or there can be coma, but there will also be concomitant symptoms of high fever, agitation, limb reversal, and crimson tongue. In most cases, pathogenic *qì* has entered deeply into the construction and blood aspects. Phlegm covering results from damp-heat fermenting into phlegm and covering the clear orifice. The subsequent loss of consciousness is not very deep. There are symptoms such as intermittent delirious speech, intermittent clouding of the spirit, and thick yellow slimy moss all over the tongue. When this is seen, it is usually seen in damp warmth diseases.

Clouded spirit with delirious speech can also result from *qì* aspect stomach and intestine repletion heat, or blood amassing in the lower burner. During *qì* aspect gastrointestinal repletion heat, there are normally accompanying symptoms of high fever and thirst, or abdominal distention with pain that refuses pressure, and constipation. In other words, there are normally *yáng* brightness internal repletion heat patterns. But when blood amasses in the lower burner there are generally symptoms of hard fullness in the lower abdomen, black-colored stools, and mania. This pattern indicates obstructing and stagnating of static blood.

I. TETANIC REVERSAL*

Tetany refers to severe muscular contraction. Clinically, it is expressed as spasms of the extremities, clenched jaw, upward-staring eyes, and neck spasms or in severe cases arched-back rigidity. Reversal (in this case) means loss of consciousness.

---

*The term "reversal (*jué*)" is an abbreviation for "reversal pattern" (i.e., *jué zhèng* 厥證). Reversal pattern can mean: 1. Unconsciousness. 2. Coldness of the four limbs. 3. Critical dysuria. In warm diseases reversal usually means unconsciousness or cold limbs.

Tetany and reversal are different symptoms, but if seen during the course of a warm disease they either occur concurrently or one follows the other—either tetany occurs and is later followed by reversal, or reversal occurs and is later followed by tetany. For this reason these two symptoms are normally considered together and referred to as "tetanic reversal." Tetanic reversal that appears during a warm disease is a characteristic reflection of liver wind stirring internally. Since the liver is the viscera of wind and wood, and since it governs the sinew vessels, both blazing of warm disease pathogenic heat and vacuity of *yīn* essence can evoke movement of liver wind and cause sinew vessel contractions. Accordingly, in clinical practice, tetanic reversal can be divided into vacuity and repletion types.

Internal movement of replete wind occurs when flaring heat pathogens move liver wind, and liver wind fans fire, creating a vicious circle. It occurs, in short, when "extreme heat engenders wind." Usually, if this takes place during a warm disease, it does so during the heat-abundant stage. The main expressions are convulsions that come on with great force and continue unabated for indefinite periods, clenched jaw, neck spasms or in severe cases arched-back rigidity, upward-staring of eyes, cold limbs, clouded spirit, and delirious speech. The pulse is usually surging and rapid or string-like and rapid with force and the tongue is red or crimson. When these symptoms appear, they indicate that the condition is already critical. Clinical experience shows that the frequency and duration of tetanic reversal is related to prognosis.

Internal stirring of vacuity wind occurs when heat pathogens lodge for prolonged periods, consume and injure the *yīn* fluids, and cause the sinew vessels to lose nourishment. If this occurs in warm disease, it generally takes place during the recovery stage. Clinical expressions include slight trembling of the extremities or ticking at the corner of the lips and mild palpitations. These are manifestations of vacuity wind stirring internally. There might also be low fever, red cheeks, vexing heat in the five hearts, thin body frame, dry mouth and tongue, night sweats that cause waking, continual tiredness and desire to sleep, deafness, loss of speech, red mirror-like tongue with little moss, and fine vacuous rapid pulse. These are manifestations of severe liver and kidney true *yīn* damage. In clinical practice, it is also possible to see another type of vacuity wind moving internally, a type accompanied by damp pathogens and turbid phlegm failing to transform. In this type, vacuity harbors repletion, so for treatment to be effective, medicinal combinations must be more complex than for the more straightforward vacuity cases.

CHAPTER 6
WARM DISEASE TREATMENTS

Warm disease treatment methods are devised according to warm disease pattern identification and treatment determination theory. After using pattern identification to correctly identify formative factors and pathomechanisms, appropriate treatment methods are selected and effective formulas are chosen to eliminate pathogens and promote health by adjusting, nourishing, and supplementing physical functionings.

In warm disease pattern identification and treatment determination, treatment methods are selected according to the different types of warm heat pathogen disease factors and the defense-*qì*-construction-blood and triple burner pathological changes, as reflected by the symptoms. The externally contracted warm heat pathogens, which are the main cause of warm diseases, can be classified as wind-heat, summerheat-heat, damp-heat, and dry-heat types, according to the seasons in which they occur. At the onset of warm disease, each of these main causes generates different characteristic symptoms. So when the policy of "finding the cause in pattern differentiation; determining treatments according to causes" is applied, the different treatment methods of resolving wind and discharging heat, outthrusting the exterior and clearing summerheat, diffusing the exterior and transforming dampness, and coursing the exterior and moisturizing dryness can be selected as appropriate. Despite their differing formative factors, as the warm diseases of the four seasons develop, their pathomechanic transformations are always limited to the defense-*qì*-construction-blood and triple burner systems. In clinical practice, suitable treatments are determined by observing their different symptom expressions, analyzing their pathomechanisms, and correctly identifying their disease types. As Yè Tiān Shì said:

> *When pathogens are in the defense, the treatment is to promote sweating. When pathogens are in the qì, the treatment is to clear qì. When pathogens are in the construction, the treatment is to outthrust heat and transfer qì. And when pathogens are in the blood, consuming and stirring the blood, the treatment must be to urgently cool and dissipate the blood.*

Wú Jú Tōng said:

> *Treatments [for the] upper burner [must be] mist-like [i.e., upbearing medicinals must be used]; treatments [for the] middle burner [must be] balance-like [ie., harmonizing medicinals must be used]; treatments [for the] lower burner [must be] authority-like [i.e., downbearing medicinals must be used].*

These passages concisely specify the appropriate policies for treating different defense-*qì*-construction-blood and triple burner patterns. Since all warm disease treatments are planned and administered according to the results of pattern identification, no matter what the disease, each treatment method can always be applied to the symptom pattern for which it was devised. Conversely, different treatment methods are used for different clinical expressions, even in a single warm disease. In other words, as a matter of policy, same patterns are treated with same methods, and different patterns with different methods. This is a succinct implementation of pattern identification and treatment determination.

The main warm disease treatment methods are selected according to "defense-*qì*-construction-blood and triple burner pattern identification," "finding the cause in pattern differentiation" and "determining treatments according to causes." They include the exterior-resolving, heat-clearing, harmonizing, dampness-transforming, downward-throughclearing, construction-clearing, blood-cooling, orifice-opening, wind-extinguishing, *yīn*-nourishing, and desertion-stemming methods. In this chapter, a separate discussion is devoted to each.

I. THE EXTERIOR-RESOLVING METHOD

Resolving the exterior means eliminating exterior pathogens, and the exterior-resolving method is the treatment method used to eliminate them. Its functions are to course and discharge the interstices and to chase pathogens outward. Since the use of this method normally results in the coursing through of skin and hair and the induction of sweating that discharges pathogens from the exterior, it is sometimes also called the sweating method. In clinical practice, it is generally used during the initial stages of a warm disease, for external patterns with defense-aspect pathogens. But just as there are several different types of warm disease pathogens, including wind-heat, summerheat-heat, damp-heat, and dry-heat, so there are several different, and corresponding, variations of the exterior-resolving method. These are listed below.

A. COURSING WIND AND DISCHARGING HEAT

This method is commonly referred to as the acrid cool exterior-resolving method. Its formulas are normally constituted of acrid scattering cooling discharging medicinals that course and scatter external-defense wind-heat pathogens. It is generally used during the initial stages of wind warmth when wind-heat attacks the lung defense causing symptoms of fever, mild aversion to cold, absence of sweating or scant sweating, mild thirst, coughing, white tongue moss, red tongue tip, and floating rapid pulse. Its paradigmatic formula is Lonicera and Forsythia Powder (*Yín Qiào Sǎn*).

B. OUTTHRUSTING THE EXTERIOR AND CLEARING SUMMERHEAT-HEAT

This method outthrusts and scatters external cold, transforms dampness, and clears summerheat. It is generally used during summer, when externally contracted summerheat-damp with cold pathogens confined to the muscle surface (i.e., summerheat-damp accompanied by cold pathogens) cause symptoms such as headache, aversion to cold, chills, fever without sweating, thirst, and vexation. Its paradigmatic formula is Newly Supplemented Elsholtzia Beverage (*Xīn Jiā Xiāng Rú Yǐn*).

C. DIFFUSING THE EXTERIOR AND TRANSFORMING DAMPNESS

This is a method in which aromatic, diffusing, outthrusting medicinals are used to course and transform dampness at the muscle surface. It is therefore prescribed during the initial stages of damp warmth, when damp pathogens encumber and obstruct the muscle surface causing symptoms such as aversion to cold, [subjective feelings of] heavy body, fever, scant sweating, slimy white tongue moss, and soggy, moderate pulse. Its paradigmatic formula is Modified Agastache Qì-Righting Powder (*Huò Xiāng Zhèng Qì Sǎn*).

D. COURSING THE EXTERIOR AND MOISTURIZING DRYNESS

This is a method in which acrid cooling clearing moisturizing medicinals are used to course and resolve lung defense dry-heat pathogens. It is usually prescribed for dry-heat damaging the lung with symptoms such as headache, fever, coughing with little expectoration, sore dry throat, dry nose and lips, white tongue moss, red tongue tip, and insufficient tongue fluids. Its paradigmatic formula is Mulberry Leaf and Apricot Kernel Decoction (*Sāng Xìng Tāng*).

When using the above four methods in clinical practice, variations are made according to accompanying symptoms. It can be appropriate, for example, to nourish *yīn* and resolve the exterior, boost *qì* and resolve the exterior, resolve the exterior and clear the interior, resolve the exterior and outthrust rashes, or course the exterior and resolve toxins.

When considering the use of the exterior-resolving method, both of the following cautions must be observed. Firstly, since exterior-resolving wind-cold-scattering prescriptions assist transformation of heat into fire, not only is their usage contraindicated in warm diseases with external heat patterns, but it is also restricted when "cold envelops fire." Although small quantities of acrid exterior-resolving medicinals can be used in patterns of "cold enveloping fire," they should be used for short periods only. Secondly, when the exterior-resolving method is being used, unless treatment is discontinued at the appropriate time, too much sweating damages fluids.

II. THE QÌ-CLEARING METHOD

This method clears and discharges *qì* aspect heat pathogens. It has heat-clearing, fire-draining, and *qì*-dynamic-diffusing functions, so when administered it normally relieves fever, preserves liquid, eliminates vexation, and stops thirst. In clinical practice, it is generally used for heat in the *qì* aspect (i.e., internal heat patterns). Since heat pathogens cause warm diseases and "cold treats heat," warm diseases commonly create conditions in which the *qì*-clearing method may be used. Provided there are no signs of internal binding and repletion, or pathogenic heat entering the construction or blood, it may be used whenever external pathogens enter internally. The *qì*-clearing method is subdivided into several different types according to its different accompanying functions. These are as follows.

A. MILDLY CLEARING AND DIFFUSING *QÌ*

This is a method in which mild clearing medicinals are used to outthrust heat and discharge pathogens, and diffuse and free the *qì* dynamic. It is generally used after the initial transference of warm disease pathogens into the *qì* aspect, when heat that is not yet very strong and loss of diffusing and freeing function cause symptoms of fever, mild thirst, anguish in the heart, and thin yellow tongue moss. Its paradigmatic formula is Supplemented Gardenia and Fermented Soybean Decoction (*Zhī Chǐ Tāng Jiā Wèi*).

B. CLEARING *QÌ* WITH COLD AND ACRIDITY

This is a method in which acrid cold medicinals are used to clear *qì* aspect heat pathogens. It is normally used when strong heat in the *yáng* brightness *qì* aspect causes symptoms of vigorous fever, great sweating, vexation, thirst, dry yellow tongue moss, and surging rapid pulse. Its paradigmatic formula is White Tiger Decoction (*Bái Hǔ Tāng*).

C. CLEARING HEAT AND DRAINING FIRE

This is a method in which bitter cold medicinals are used to directly clear internal heat, and to clear and discharge pathogenic fire. Its principal application is for smoldering heat confined in the *qì* aspect that transforms into fire and causes symptoms of lingering fever, vexation and agitation, bitter taste in the mouth, thirst, dark yellow urine, red tongue, and yellow tongue moss. Its paradigmatic formula is Coptis Toxin-Resolving Decoction (*Huáng Lián Jiě Dú Tāng*).

The *qì*-clearing method has a wide range of applications and a wide range of modifications. Its major uses are as follows:

1. It is used to diffuse *qì* and outthrust the exterior. In this application, mildly clearing *qì*-diffusing medicinals are combined with exterior outthrusting medicinals to treat the initial stage of heat transferring into the *qì* aspect (before the external patterns have resolved).

2. It is used to clear heat and nourish *yīn*. In this application, *qì*-clearing heat-discharging medicinals are combined with liquid-engendering humor-nourishing medicinals to treat patterns of strong *qì* aspect heat with damaged *yīn* fluid.

3. It is used to clear heat and diffuse the lungs. In this application, *qì*-clearing heat-discharging medicinals are combined with lung diffusing lung *qì* downbearing medicinals, mainly to treat smoldering heat in the lungs with secondary patterns of lung *qì* confinement and closure.

4. It is used to clear heat and resolve toxins. In this application heat-clearing fire-draining medicinals are combined with toxin-resolving swelling-dispersing medicinals to treat smoldering and binding of heat toxins accompanied by scorching hot painful red swellings at certain limited areas.

When considering the use of the *qì*-clearing method, the following cautions must be observed.

1. The *qì*-clearing method cannot be used until after warm disease external patterns have resolved. The abuse of cold and cooling medicinals causes "freezing" and concealment of disease pathogens rather than their resolution.

2. Cold and cooling *qì*-clearing medicinals are contraindicated when damp-heat is lingering in the *qì* aspect. If used erroneously they obstruct and conceal disease pathogens.

3. Great care must be exercised when using the *qì*-clearing method on patients with pre-existing *yáng* vacuity.

III. THE HARMONIZING AND RESOLVING METHOD

"Harmonizing" is one of the eight treatment methods. It has harmonizing-resolving and coursing-discharging functions. Whenever warm disease pathogens are neither externally nor internally bound—whenever they are, for example, confined in lesser *yáng*, lodged in the triple burner, or concealed in the membrane source, this method can be used to outthrust pathogenic heat and to diffuse and clear the *qì* dynamic. It aims to resolve the exterior and harmonize the interior. Its various subdivisions are discussed below.

A. CLEARING AND DISCHARGING LESSER *YÁNG*

This method is used primarily to clear and discharge half-external half-internal lesser *yáng* pathogenic heat, but can also be used to transform phlegm and harmonize the stomach. Its principal application is for heat confined in lesser *yáng* with failure of the harmonizing and descending functions of the stomach—for symptoms such as alternating fevers and chills, bitter taste in the mouth, rib-side pain, strong thirst, dark yellow urine, stomach duct dilations, nausea, slimy yellow tongue moss, red tongue, and string-like rapid pulse. Its paradigmatic formula is Sweet Wormwood and Scutellaria Gallbladder-Clearing Decoction (*Hāo Qín Qīng Dǎn Tāng*).

B. SCATTERING, DISPERSING, PENETRATING, AND DISCHARGING

This method is used to scatter and disperse triple burner *qì* aspect pathogens by diffusing the *qì* dynamic, and by discharging and transforming phlegm-heat. It is generally administered when pathogens lodge in the triple burner and failure of *qì* transformation leads to turbid phlegm obstruction with symptoms such as appearing and disappearing fevers and chills, chest dilations, abdominal distention, scant urine, and slimy tongue moss. Its paradigmatic prescription is Gallbladder-Warming Decoction (*Wēn Dǎn Tāng*) with modifications, but commonly used medicinal combinations such as apricot kernel (*xìng rén*), magnolia bark (*hòu pò*), and poria (*fú líng*) are also illustrative.

C. MEMBRANE SOURCE OPENING AND EXTENDING

This is a method in which turbid damp pathogens are coursed, disinhibited, and outthrust from the membrane source, so it is used primarily for turbid damp-heat confined in and blocking the *qì* aspect (i.e., for "pathogens concealed in the membrane source"). In cases like these, where there are symptoms such as more chills and less fevers, stomach duct dilations, abdominal distention, slimy white tongue moss that looks like powder piled on the tongue, and crimson tongue, formulas such as Léi's Membrane Source Diffusing and Outthrusting Method (*Léi Shì Xuān Tòu Mó Yuán Fǎ*) are generally used.

In clinical practice, the harmonizing and resolving method is normally combined with other methods according to the condition. It can, for instance, be combined with the heat-clearing dampness-transforming method, or the gallbladder-disinhibiting yellowness-abating method.

When considering the use of this method, the following cautions must be observed:

1. Although the lesser *yáng* clearing and discharging method can outthrust pathogens and discharge heat, its heat-clearing function is not very strong. It is inappropriate when patients have strong internal heat.

2. Although the scattering, dispersing, penetrating, and discharging method and the membrane source opening and extending method are both better than the lesser *yáng* clearing and discharging method at coursing and transforming turbid dampness, they cannot be used when heat is half external and half internal.

IV. THE DAMPNESS-DISPELLING METHOD

This is a method wherein medicinals that are aromatic and dampness-transforming, bitter and warm drying, dampness-eliminating, and bland and dampness-disinhibiting are used to dry damp pathogens. Its actions are to diffuse and throughclear the *qì* dynamic, to promote the transforming function of the spleen and harmonize the stomach, to throughclear and disinhibit the water-path, and to transform dampness and discharge turbidity. In clinical practice, it is normally prescribed when warm diseases are marked by prominent damp-heat. It is subdivided, according to its clinical functions, into the following sections.

A. DIFFUSING *QÌ* AND TRANSFORMING DAMPNESS

This method diffuses and throughclears the *qì* dynamic, and outthrusts and transforms damp pathogens. It is normally used during the initial stage of damp warmth, when fermenting dampness engenders heat that confines and obstructs the *qì* dynamic. In such cases there are symptoms of fever that intensifies during the afternoon, sweating that fails to eliminate fever or mild aversion to cold, oppression in the chest, stomach duct dilations, scant urine, slimy white tongue moss, and soggy, moderate pulse. Its paradigmatic formula is Three Kernels Decoction (*Sān Rén Tāng*).

B. DRYING DAMPNESS AND DISCHARGING HEAT

This is a method in which acrid-opening bitter-descending combinations are used to dry dampness and discharge heat. It is generally prescribed when damp warmth dampness which is gradually transforming into heat becomes trapped and concealed in the middle burner, causing symptoms such as fever, thirst but little desire to drink, stomach duct dilations, abdominal distention, nausea, and slimy yellow tongue moss. Its paradigmatic formula is Wang's Coptis and Magnolia Bark Beverage (*Wáng Shì Lián Pò Yǐn*).

C. SCATTERING AND DISINHIBITING DAMP PATHOGENS

This is a method in which bland drying medicinals that disinhibit urine and drain dampness are used to eliminate pathogens via urine. It is generally prescribed when lower burner blockages that result from dampness harboring smoldering heat cause symptoms such as scant urine or even complete blockage of urine, sensations of heat steaming up to the head with subjective feelings of head distention, white tongue moss, and thirst. Its paradigmatic formula is Poria Skin Decoction (*Fú Líng Pí Tāng*).

Although there are circumstances in which each of the above three methods may be correctly prescribed in isolation, in clinical practice they are normally used in combinations. The *qì*-diffusing dampness-transforming method is, for example, normally combined with the dampness-scattering dampness-disinhibiting method, whereas the dampness-drying heat-discharging method is generally used with the *qì*-diffusing dampness-transforming method. Moreover, dampness-dispelling methods are also commonly combined with heat-clearing methods, yellowness-abating methods, stomach-harmonizing methods, and coursing and dispelling methods according to the patient's condition.

When considering the use of the dampness-dispelling method the following cautions must be observed:

1. If dampness has already transformed into dryness, dampness-dispelling methods are contraindicated.

2. If a patient's *yīn* fluids are insufficient, the dampness-dispelling method must be used cautiously.

V. THE DOWNWARD-THROUGHCLEARING METHOD

This method courses and abducts internal repletion and discharges below to expel pathogens. Its actions are to throughclear stools, to drain pathogenic heat, to flush accumulations and stagnations, and to throughclear blood stasis and break binds. It is therefore suitable for internal binding of replete pathogens with form (i.e., conditions like heat bind in the intestinal bowel creating gastrointestinal accumulations and stagnations), and for blood amassing in the lower burner. It is subdivided into the following sections according to its clinical functions.

A. THROUGHCLEARING BOWELS AND DISCHARGING HEAT

This is a method in which bitter cold downbearing medicinals are used to drain repletion heat from the intestinal bowels. It is normally prescribed when heat transfers to *yáng* brightness and binds internally in the intestinal bowels, causing symptoms such as tidal fever, delirious speech, constipation, abdominal distention that feels very hard and refuses pressure, old yellow tongue moss or in severe cases scorched-black tongue moss with thorns, and sunken replete pulse. Its paradigmatic formulas are Greater Qì-Infusing Decoction (*Dà Chéng Qì Tāng*) and Stomach-Regulating Qì-Infusing Decoction (*Tiáo Wèi Chéng Qì Tāng*).

B. COURSING STAGNATION AND THROUGHCLEARING STOOLS

This method not only throughclears and courses accumulations and stagnations, but also discharges confined heat below. It is generally used for accumulations and stagnations of damp-heat that combine and bind in the stomach and intestines, causing symptoms such as dilations and fullness in the gastroabdominal region, nausea and vomiting, turbid yellow-brown diarrhea, and yellow tongue moss. Its paradigmatic formula is Unripe Bitter Orange Stagnation-Abducting Decoction (*Zhǐ Shí Dǎo Zhì Tāng*).

C. THROUGHCLEARING STASIS AND BREAKING BINDS

This method breaks and scatters lower burner blood stasis amassment and binding by downward-throughclearing, and is generally prescribed when blood amassment in the lower burner results from stasis and heat binding together during a warm disease. It is used for symptoms of distention fullness and acute pain in the lower abdomen, constipation yet normal urination, manic behavior, rinsing of the mouth but no desire to drink, crimson-purple tongue, and fine replete pulse. Its paradigmatic formula is Peach Kernel Qì-Infusing Decoction (*Táo Rén Chéng Qì Tāng*).

The downward-throughclearing method, particularly the bitter cold downward-throughclearing method, is one of the most effective methods for treating warm diseases. Liǔ Bǎo Yí (柳寶詒) pointed out its importance when he explained:

> *The stomach is the sea of the five viscera and the six bowels; it occupies the middle earth, and it readily collects and stores. Therefore, pathogenic heat that enters the stomach does not transfer. When warm disease heat binds in the stomach bowel, the downward-throughclearing method yields results in 60 to 70 percent of all cases. . . . Premature downward-throughclearing is not a serious mistake in a warm disease.*

Of course in clinical practice, different modifications are made according to different patient conditions. It is, for example, quite common for both the downward-throughclearing and reinforcing methods to be used together. The simultaneous use of the downward-throughclearing and right-*qì*-assisting method is a widespread practice, suitable for *yáng* brightness bowel repletions with right *qì* vacuity. In bowel repletion accompanied by *yīn* fluid vacuity, the downward-throughclearing method is combined with the *yīn*-nourishing method. Also, downward-throughclearing can be combined with lung-diffusing, orifice-opening, or six-bowel clearing and coursing to treat *yáng* brightness bowel repletions with phlegm-heat obstructing the lung, pathogens blocking the pericardium, or binding of small intestine heat.

When considering the use of the downward-throughclearing method the following cautions must be observed.

1. This method is contraindicated in cases of repletion where warm disease pathogens have already transferred to the interior but internal binding has not occurred (i.e., where pathogenic heat or damp-heat is without form).

2. It must be used cautiously when right *qì* is vacuous and weak. When, for example, the pathogens are replete and the right *qì* is vacuous, this method must be combined with the reinforcing method.

3. Since constipation that develops during the final stage of a warm disease occurs because the fluids are desiccated and the intestines are drying out, the bitter cold downward-throughclearing method is contraindicated.

VI. THE CONSTRUCTION-CLEARING METHOD

The construction-clearing method, a subcategory of the clearing method of the eight methods, is used to clear and discharge construction aspect heat pathogens. Its functions are to clear construction, discharge heat, and nourish construction-*yīn*. In clinical practice, it is prescribed for construction aspect patterns where pathogens have entered the construction but have not yet stirred the blood.

A. CLEARING CONSTRUCTION AND DISCHARGING HEAT

This is a method in which medicinals that clear and resolve construction aspect heat pathogens are used in combination with light clearing outthrusting discharging medicinals. It induces transference of pathogenic *qì* from the construction to the *qì* aspect and then resolves it. It is prescribed when heat enters the construction aspect causing symptoms such as fever that intensifies at night, vexation, insomnia, perhaps delirious speech, rashes that have only partially surfaced, and crimson tongue. Its paradigmatic formula is Construction-Clearing Decoction (*Qīng Yíng Tāng*).

B. CLEARING BOTH *QÌ* AND CONSTRUCTION

This is a method in which construction-clearing medicinals and *qì*-clearing medicinals are coupled. It is used for pathogens entering the construction with *qì* heat remaining exuberant (i.e., for patterns of intensifying of heat at both the *qì* and construction). In such cases there are symptoms of vigorous fever, strong thirst, vexation, macula spots that have surfaced to the exterior, crimson tongue, and dry yellow tongue moss. Generally, formulas like Jade Lady Variant Brew (*Jiā Jiǎn Yù Nǚ Jiān*) are prescribed.

In clinical practice, the construction-clearing method is usually coupled with the *qì*-clearing method. But depending on the patient's condition, it sometimes needs to be coupled with other methods, such as the orifice-opening method or the wind-extinguishing method.

Before using the construction-clearing method the following cautions must be observed:

1. Even though internal heat may be very strong, if the pathogen has lodged in the *qì* aspect, without having entered the construction aspect, this method is contraindicated—if used erroneously it guides deep entry of pathogenic *qì*.

2. When pathogens have first entered the construction but not yet stirred the blood, they cannot be successfully transferred to the *qì* aspect and be resolved solely by using medicinals that clear and cool the construction-blood. Medicinals that outthrust and discharge

must also be used. Even when pathogens have entered the blood, the sole use of construction-clearing heat-discharging medicinals will not be successful—they must be immediately supplemented with medicinals that cool and medicinals that dissipate the blood.

VII. THE BLOOD-COOLING METHOD

This is a method in which clearing and cooling medicinals are used to clear and disperse blood aspect heat toxin pathogens. Its functions are to cool blood and nourish *yīn*, clear fire and resolve toxins, throughclear the network vessels, and scatter blood. It is used principally when warm disease pathogenic heat enters deeply into the blood aspect, causing strong heat toxins, damaged network vessels, and stirring blood patterns. In clinical practice, it is subdivided into the following two methods.

A. COOLING AND SCATTERING BLOOD

This method cools and resolves blood aspect heat pathogens, quickens blood, and scatters blood. It is suitable for use when heat enters the blood aspect and exuberant heat stirs the blood. In such cases, there are symptoms such as scorching heat, agitation or in severe cases mania, delirious speech, vomiting of blood, nose bleeding, blood in the stools, blood in the urine, concentrated rashes, and dark-crimson tongue. Its paradigmatic formula is Rhinoceros Horn and Rehmannia Decoction (*Xī Jiǎo Dì Huáng Tāng*).

B. CLEARING *QÌ* AND BLOOD WITH LARGE [DOSES]

This is a method in which large doses of heat-clearing toxin-resolving medicinals are used to clear and disperse *qì* and blood aspect triple burner heat toxins. Its principal application is for congested exuberant warm disease heat toxins that force *qì* and blood to overflow and spread through the triple burner, causing symptoms such as vigorous fever, stabbing headache, thirst with desire to drink cold drinks, foul mouth odor, visual distortion, delirious speech, mania, bone and joint aches, backache in which the back feels like it has been dealt a crushing blow, purple-black rashes or nosebleeds or blood in the urine, dry yellow or scorched-black tongue moss, and purple tongue. Its paradigmatic prescription is Scourge-Clearing Toxin-Vanquishing Beverage (*Qīng Wēn Bài Dú Yǐn*).

The blood-cooling method is normally combined with the orifice-opening method, the wind-extinguishing method, or the blood-quickening stasis-transforming method.

When considering the use of the blood-cooling method the following cautions must be observed:

1. Even after heat has entered the construction aspect, unless it is stirring the blood, it is still too early to use the blood-cooling method.

2. When non-stop bleeding results after intensifying of blood heat causes stasis and stagnation in the network vessels, blood-quickening stasis-scattering medicinals must be used without delay.

3. When warm disease heat toxins force overflowing internally and externally, above and below, thinking must not be limited by defense-*qì*-construction-blood theory. In such cases, large doses of clearing and resolving medicinals must be used to strongly clear the *qì* and blood, drain the fire, and resolve the toxins.

VIII. THE ORIFICE-OPENING METHOD

This treatment method clears the mind by opening and clearing through the heart orifices. Its functions are to clear the heart and transform phlegm, to outthrust the network vessels with aromatic medicinals, and to open closures and throughclear the orifices. It is generally used when warm disease pathogens close the pericardium and cloud the spirit or cause coma. In clinical practice, it is subdivided into the following two sections.

A. CLEARING THE HEART AND OPENING THE ORIFICES

This method clarifies the mind by clearing and discharging pathogenic heat from the pericardium, and by transforming phlegm and outthrusting the network vessels. It is used when warm disease heat counterflows into the pericardium and blocks the heart orifices, creating symptoms such as scorching hot body with limb reversal (i.e., cold limbs), clouded spirit with delirious speech or coma without speech, sluggish tongue, and vivid-crimson tongue. Its most commonly used formulas include Peaceful Palace Bovine Bezoar Pill (*Ān Gōng Niú Huáng Wán*), Supreme Jewel Elixir (*Zhì Bǎo Dān*), and Purple Snow Elixir (*Zǐ Xuě Dān*).

B. SWEEPING PHLEGM AND OPENING THE ORIFICES

This method diffuses the orifices and opens closures by clearing and transforming both damp-heat and turbid phlegm. It is suitable for use when confined steaming damp-heat ferments into turbid phlegm, which clouds the mind and closes the clear orifices, causing symptoms such as clouded spirit (the mind being sometimes clear and sometimes confused), periods of delirious speech, red tongue, and sticky slimy yellow moss. Its paradigmatic formula is Acorus and Curuma Decoction (*Chāng Pú Yù Jīn Tāng*).

The orifice-opening method is used during emergencies to alleviate clouded spirit. Clinically, it is almost always used with supplementary methods. The heart-clearing orifice-opening method, for example, is normally used with the construction-clearing, blood-cooling, wind-extinguishing, or desertion-stemming method, while the phlegm-sweeping orifice-opening method is normally used with the heat-clearing or dampness-transforming method.

Before using the orifice-opening method the following cautions must be observed:

1. When clouded spirit is attributable to exuberant *qì* aspect heat, the orifice-opening method is contraindicated.

2. Even when pathogens enter the construction-blood, unless they cause closure and reversal, the heart-clearing orifice-opening method cannot be used.

3. The functions of the heart-clearing orifice-opening method and the phlegm-sweeping orifice-opening method are different (i.e., when used clinically, they are used for different patterns so they must not be confused).

4. Since in the treatment of warm diseases, the orifice-opening method is used as an emergency measure, the appropriate supplementary methods must be determined according to the relative strength and weakness of the right and pathogenic *qì*, as reflected in the clinical expressions.

IX. THE WIND-EXTINGUISHING METHOD

This is the method used to extinguish liver wind and control tetanic reversal. Its functions are to settle fright and stop tetanic spasms. In warm disease, it is prescribed for internal stirring of liver wind with convulsions or tetanic reversals, and in clinical practice it is subdivided into the following two sections.

A. COOLING THE LIVER AND EXTINGUISHING WIND

This method acts principally to clear heat and cool the liver, extinguish wind, and stop tetanic spasms. It is suitable for use when intensifying of warm disease heat pathogens stir liver wind internally causing symptoms of scorching body heat and limb reversal (i.e., cold limbs), intermittent tetanic spasms of the arms and legs, and in severe cases arched-back rigidity, clouded spirit without speech, and string-like rapid pulse. Its paradigmatic prescription is Antelope Horn and Uncaria Decoction (*Líng Jiǎo Guō Téng Tāng*).

B. NOURISHING *YĪN* AND EXTINGUISHING WIND

This method extinguishes vacuity wind by fostering *yīn* and subduing *yáng*. It is suitable for use during the late stages of warm disease when the true *yīn* is depleted and damaged, the liver looses nourishment, and vacuity wind stirs internally—when there are symptoms such as trembling of the hands and feet or in severe cases convulsions, limb reversal, lassitude of the spirit, crimson tongue, scant tongue moss, and vacuous fine pulse. Its paradigmatic formula is Major Wind-Stabilizing Pill (*Dà Dìng Fēng Zhū*).

The wind-extinguishing method is suitable for treating tetanic reversals, but in clinical practice is seldom used alone. Depending on the nature of the pathogen, the liver-cooling wind-extinguishing method is normally combined with the *qì*-clearing, construction-clearing, blood-cooling, or downward-throughclearing method, whereas the *yīn*-nourishing wind-extinguishing method is normally combined with the *qì*-boosting, desertion-stemming, blood-quickening, or phlegm-transforming method.

When considering the use of the wind-extinguishing method, the following issues must be considered.

1. The liver-cooling wind-extinguishing and the *yīn*-nourishing wind-extinguishing methods are very different. In the former, the focus is on eliminating the pathogens; in the latter, on assisting the right *qì*. Clinically, therefore, distinctions must be made as to whether moving wind is replete or vacuous.

2. Even though children who are suffering from warm diseases with pathogens in the defense and *qì* aspects generally develop convulsions very quickly (due to their high fever), the principal treatment is still to clear the heat and outthrust the pathogens. As soon as their fevers reduce, their convulsions recede. Liver-cooling wind-extinguishing medicinals must not be used too early.

X. THE *YĪN*-NOURISHING METHOD

This method nourishes and supplements *yīn* humor. Since its main functions are to nourish and supplement true *yīn*, to engender liquid and nourish humor, and to moisten dryness and control fire, it is generally used when warm disease heat pathogens are gradually resolving and *yīn* humor is damaged. Warm disease heat pathogens can easily detriment and damage fluids (being particularly liable to damage liquid and consume humor during the final stages of a disease), and the degree of damage to the *yīn* humor is closely related to the patient's prognosis. The medical experts of ancient times therefore postulated, "For one part fluid there is one part engendering-dynamic." As this suggests, the *yīn*-nourishing method is commonly used in the treatment of warm diseases. This method is subdivided into the following three sections, according to its different clinical functions.

A. NOURISHING THE LUNGS AND STOMACH

This is a method in which sweet cold moisturizing medicinals are used to nourish lung and stomach fluids. It is suitable for use when heat damages stomach *yīn* humor and then begins to gradually resolve, leaving symptoms such as mouth, nose, lip, and throat desiccation, dry coughing with scant phlegm, and dry tongue moss. Its paradigmatic formula is Adenophora/Glehnia and Ophiopogon Decoction (*Shā Shēn Mài Mén Dōng Tāng*).

B. INCREASING HUMOR AND MOISTURIZING THE INTESTINES

This is a method in which sweet cold and salty cold medicinals are used to engender liquid and nourish humor, moisten the intestines, and throughclear stools. It is generally used when heat pathogens damage *yīn* humor, desiccate liquid, dry the intestines, and then begins to gradually resolve, leaving symptoms such as constipation, dry mouth and throat, and dry red tongue. Its paradigmatic formula is Humor-Increasing Decoction (*Zēng Yè Tāng*).

C. NOURISHING AND SUPPLEMENTING KIDNEY *YĪN*

This is a method in which sweet cold nourishing-moisturizing medicinals are used to supplement true *yīn*, strengthen water, and subdue *yáng*. It is generally prescribed when lingering warm heat pathogens rob and scorch the true *yīn*, creating increased vacuity diminished pathogen patterns with symptoms such as fever, red complexion, more heat in the palms and soles than in the back of the hands and top of the feet, dry mouth and throat, lassitude of the spirit, desire to sleep, sometimes palpitations, crimson tongue with scant moss, and a vacuous, fine or bound, regularly-interrupted pulse. Its paradigmatic formula is Pulse Restorative Variant Decoction (*Jiā Jiǎn Fù Mài Tāng*).

The functions of Pulse Restorative Variant Decoction (*Jiā Jiǎn Fù Mài Tāng*) are to nourish the *yīn* and reinforce the blood, clear the heat, and restore the pulse. It is used to treat conditions that occur after warm heat diseases, in which residual pathogenic heat lingers and yin-fluids are damaged (hence increased vacuity diminished pathogen patterns).

The *yīn*-nourishing method has a wide range of applications in the treatment of warm diseases, and can therefore be used in combination with a wide range of other treatment methods. It can be appropriate, for example, to nourish *yīn* and resolve the exterior, nourish *yīn* and clear heat, nourish *yīn* and downward throughclear, or nourish *yīn* and extinguish wind.

When considering the use of the *yīn*-nourishing method, the following contraindications and cautions must be observed.

1. It is contraindicated whenever warm disease pathogenic heat is exuberant, because if used erroneously it causes the pathogen to lodge.

2. It must be used with due caution whenever damp-heat patterns are being treated. If not used cautiously, pathogens become adhesive and very difficult to resolve.

XI. THE DESERTION-SECURING METHOD

This is an emergency rectification measure used for vacuity desertion. It includes the *yáng*-returning counterflow-stemming method and the *qì*-boosting desertion-securing method. In clinical practice, it is generally prescribed for the critical conditions of *yáng* collapse reversal counterflow and sudden desertion of right *qì*. Even though *yīn* vacuity occurs quite commonly in warm diseases, the unusual changes of *yáng* collapse and *qì* desertion do not normally follow. They generally eventuate only if the *yīn* has been suddenly damaged during the development of a disease—a predicament that can be caused by either vacuity of right *qì* with overabundance of pathogenic *qì*, or abuse of sweat-inducing and downward-throughclearing methods. In such cases the situation is critical, so the *yáng*-returning counterflow-stemming method or the *qì*-boosting desertion-stemming method must be used. These two methods are discussed below.

A. BOOSTING *QÌ* AND SECURING DESERTION

This method boosts *qì* and engenders liquid, stops sweating and secures desertion. It is normally used when, during the course of a warm disease, the *qì* and *yīn* have both been damaged and the right *qì* is verging on desertion—when there are symptoms such as great sweating, shortness of breath, lassitude of the spirit, physical tiredness, and fine pulse without strength. Its paradigmatic formula is Pulse-Engendering Powder (*Shēng Mài Sǎn*).

B. RETURNING *YÁNG* AND STEMMING COUNTERFLOW

This is a method in which acrid hot medicinals are used to rouse *yáng*. It is generally used for sudden desertion of *yáng qì* with symptoms of cold extremities, dribbling sweat, expiration of spirit, curled-up posture, white complexion, and fine faint pulse that has nearly expired. Its paradigmatic formula is Ginseng, Aconite, Dragon Bone, and Oyster Shell Decoction (*Shēn Fù Lóng Mǔ Tāng*).

In clinical practice, the above two methods are normally used together. For internal closure with external desertion they are generally coupled with orifice-opening methods.

When considering the use of the desertion-stemming method, the following cautions must be observed:

1. The desertion-stemming method is normally used only in critical conditions, so when used it must be used without delay. Also, the number of doses per day, the time between doses, and the strength of doses must be understood. Likewise, the patient's changing condition needs to be followed so that beneficial modifications can be made.

2. Since the desertion-stemming method is one of the emergency treatment methods, it must be used when appropriate and then discontinued immediately. As soon as the *yáng* returns and the desertion stops, pattern identification and treatment determination must be performed according to the patient's condition.

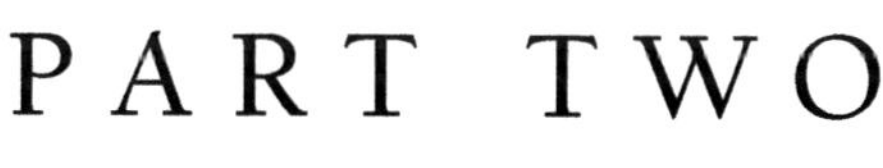

PART TWO

CHAPTER 7
WIND WARMTH

Wind warmth is an externally contracted hot disease that results from attacks by pathogenic wind-heat. It is marked, initially, by characteristic lung defense symptoms of fever, slight aversion to wind or cold, headache, coughing, and slight thirst, and it usually occurs during spring or winter. If it occurs during spring it is called wind warmth, and if it occurs during winter, winter warmth. As Chén Píng Bó (陳平伯) wrote:

> *Winter wind diseases usually occur in spring and winter, with or without aversion to wind, but always with fever, coughing, and unquenchable thirst.*

This passage not only concurs with the assertion that wind warmth occurs during spring and winter, but (except for the inconsistent symptom of unquenchable thirst) also corroborates its clinical characteristics. Wind warmth theory can be applied in pattern identification and treatment determination for biomedically defined conditions such as infectious influenza, pneumonia, and acute bronchitis.

I. DISEASE CAUSES AND PATHOLOGY

Wind warmth results when the human body is attacked by wind warmth pathogens. It can easily occur during spring, when the weather is changing from cold to warm, and people who are unable to acclimatize or who have poor resistance are attacked by pathogenic *qì*. It can also easily occur during winter, when the weather, which is normally cold, grows unseasonably warm and people are attacked by pathogenic warm wind. As Yè Tiān Shì stated, "Wind warmth attacks during spring, the qì of which is already warm." As his protegé Wú Kūn Ān (吴坤安) explained, "If the weather is fine and dry, and warm wind is too warm, attacks by its qì are called pathogenic wind warmth."

Usually, externally contracted wind-heat pathogens enter via the mouth and nose, and first damage the lung. Therefore, during the initial stages of this disease [pathological] transformations are restricted to the lung channel. The lungs govern *qì*, correspond with the defense, and tend the skin and body hair, so at the onset of the disease, lung defense symptoms generally appear. Since the right and the pathogenic *qì* are fighting, the defense *qì* fails to maintain control of its opening and closing functions. The lung *qì* is confined and therefore no longer able to diffuse, so there are symptoms of fever, aversion to wind, coughing, and thirst.

After pathogenic *qì* causes the lung defense to lose its diffusing ability, there are two ways in which the disease can develop. Firstly, it can transmit directly into the stomach. Or secondly, it can counter-transmit into the pericardium. This is why Yè Tiān Shì said, "When warm pathogens attack above, they first attack the lungs and then counter-transmit into the pericardium."

Not only does wind warmth begin by damaging the lungs, but if it transmits directly, hot pathogenic *qì* enters the stomach, and *yáng* brightness heat usually grows exuberant, or heat binds in the intestines. If it counter-transmits, it enters the pericardium, where it causes clouded spirit and delirium. During the development of this disease, when heat pathogens obstruct the lungs, instead of causing hot phlegm and rapid breathing, lung heat can enter the blood network vessels and come out as red rashes. During the final stage there can be lung and stomach *yīn* damage.

II. MAIN POINTS OF DIAGNOSIS

1. When externally contracted hot diseases occur during the seasons of winter and spring, wind warmth diseases must be considered.

2. The key criterion for diagnosis is that in the beginning there are lung defense symptoms of fever, aversion to wind, coughing, thirst, and floating pulse.

3. Although this disease and the next (i.e., spring warmth) both occur during the season of spring, they are different. At the beginning of wind warmth there are symptoms of external heat, but at the beginning of spring warmth there are symptoms of internal heat.

III. PATTERN IDENTIFICATION AND TREATMENT DETERMINATION

To treat this disease during its initial stage, when the pathogen is in the lung defense, use acrid cold medicinals to diffuse and resolve the exterior pathogenic *qì*. As Yè Tiān Shì recommended, "For pathogens in the defense aspect, use sweat-inducing medicinals." For transmission of pathogens into the *qì* aspect use acrid cold heat-clearing medicinals or bitter cold attacking-below medicinals. If pathogens obstruct the pericardium, then use heart-clearing orifice-opening medicinals. During the final stage, when pathogenic heat abates but lung and stomach liquid are damaged and unable to self-restore, use sweet cold clearing and nourishing medicinals to treat the lung and stomach *yīn*.

A. THE DISEASE PATTERN AND ITS TREATMENT IN PATHOGENS ATTACKING THE LUNG DEFENSE

Pattern

Fever, mild aversion to wind, sore throat, headache, scant sweating or absence of sweating, coughing, oppression or pain in the chest, mild thirst, thin white tongue moss, red tongue tip, and floating rapid pulse.

These symptoms are caused by wind warmth pathogens beginning to assail the lung. When pathogenic *qì* damages the exterior, defense *qì* is confined so mild aversion to wind occurs, the opening and closing function of the defense *qì* fails so scant sweating or absence of sweating occurs, the pathogenic *qì* is not resolved so heat steams upward and headache occurs, and the lung *qì* is unable to diffuse, so coughing with oppression or pain in the chest occurs.

Since wind-heat is external the tongue moss is thin and white, and the pulse is floating and rapid. And because pathogenic warm heat easily damages fluid there is mild thirst and the tongue tip is red. The symptoms of fever, mild aversion to wind, headache, scant sweating or absence of sweating, coughing, and thin white tongue moss seem much like those of externally contracted wind-cold. But in practice they are easy to differentiate because in external wind-cold the fever, which is not very high, is always accompanied by severe aversion to wind. Also, thirst is absent, and the pulse is floating and slow or floating and tight. In external wind warmth, by contrast, the fever is much higher and the aversion to wind is much less severe. Also, there is always mild thirst, and the pulse is always floating and rapid.

Treatment

Resolve the exterior with acrid-cooling medicinals; diffuse the lungs and discharge the heat.

Prescriptions

Lonicera and Forsythia Powder (*Yín Qiào Sǎn* 銀翹散)

From the Detailed Analysis of Warm Diseases (*Wēn Bìng Tiáo Biàn* 溫病條辯)

lonicera [flower] (*jīn yín huā*)	金銀花	10g
forsythia [fruit] (*lián qiào*)	連翹	10g
platycodon [root] (*jié gěng*)	桔梗	6g
arctium [seed] (*niú bàng zǐ*) (crush)	牛蒡子	10g
mint (*bò hé*) (add later)	薄荷	6g
fermented soybean (*dòu chǐ*)	豆豉	10g
schizonepeta spike (*jīng jiè*)	荊芥	12g
bamboo leaf (*dàn zhú yè*)	淡竹葉	10g
raw licorice [root] (*shēng gān cǎo*)	生甘草	6g

Grind all the medicinals into powder. Divide them into six-gram doses and boil them with fresh phragmites [root] (*xiān lú gēn*). As soon as the decoction starts giving off an aroma administer it quickly. To treat the lung, these medicinals must be kept floating and clear, so avoid boiling them for too long. If they are over-boiled their flavors become thick and enter the middle burner. If the disease is severe, administer medicinals every four hours, up to three times during the day and once at night. If the disease is mild, give every six hours, twice during the day and once at night. If the disease lingers, continue prescribing the medication.

Pathogens at the muscle exterior are treated with acrid resolving prescriptions that expel exterior pathogens. These symptoms are caused by wind warmth lodging at the exterior and must therefore be treated with the acrid cool exterior-resolving method. In the *Plain Questions: General Treatise on Essential Principles* it says, "Replete internal wind: treat with acrid cool, assist with bitter sweet flavors, and use sweet flavors to relax."

Lonicera and Forsythia Powder (*Yín Qiào Sǎn*), the paradigmatic acrid cool exterior-resolving prescription, clears and diffuses pathogens from the lung defense.

This formula contains:

§ Schizonepeta *(jīng jiè),* mint *(bò hé),* and fermented soybean *(dòu chǐ),* which promote sweating to resolve the exterior and dissipate pathogenic qì.

§ Arctium [seed] (*niú bàng zǐ*), raw licorice [root] (*shēng gān cǎo*), and platycodon [root] (*kǔ jié gěng*), which drain the lungs and stop coughing.

§ Forsythia [fruit] (*lián qiào*), lonicera [flower] (*jīn yín huā*), and bamboo leaf (*zhú yè*), which clear and diffuse heat.

§ Fresh phragmites [root] (*xiān lú gēn*), which engenders fluid and stops thirst.

Most ingredients in this prescription are acrid cool medicinals, but some are acrid and hot. Therefore, it is as Wú Jú Tōng indicated, of "average strength, acrid [and] cooling." This formula is suitable for external wind-heat with symptoms of fever, fear of cold, and absence of sweating. It is normally prepared as a powder but provided the dosages are reduced proportionally and the medicinals are not boiled for too long, it can also be prepared as a decoction.

Modifications

1. For turbid impurities obstructing the *qì* dynamic, with oppression and distention in the chest and diaphragm, add agastache (*huò xiāng*) and curcuma [tuber] (*yù jīn*) to scatter the impurities with aroma, and course and disinhibit the *qì*.

2. For thirst caused by warm heat scorching the fluids add trichosanthes root (*tiān huā fěn*) to clear heat and engender liquid.

3. For sore swollen throat caused by warm toxins add puffball (*mǎ bó*) and scrophularia [root] (*xuán shēn*) to resolve toxins and eliminate swelling.

4. For coughing caused by confined lung *qì* add apricot kernel (*xìng rén*) to disinhibit and diffuse the lung *qì*.

5. For nosebleeds caused by heat damaging the *yáng* network vessels, replace schizonepeta (*jīng jiè*) and fermented soybean (*dòu chǐ*), which are acrid and warming, with imperata [root] (*bái máo gēn*), charred biota leaf (*cè bǎi tàn*), and charred gardenia [fruit] (*zhī zǐ tàn*), which are blood-cooling and anti-bleeding.

6. For vexing sensations in the chest with dark-red tongue, caused by heat entering internally and rippling into the construction aspect, add raw rehmannia [root] (*shēng dì*) and ophiopogon [tuber] (*mài dōng*), which are heat clearing and *yīn*-nourishing.

7. For scanty dark yellow urine caused by heat damaging the fluids, add anemarrhena [root] (*zhī mǔ*), scutellaria [root] (*huáng qín*), and gardenia [fruit] (*zhī zǐ*), which are bitter and cold, plus ophiopogon [tuber] (*mài dōng*) and raw rehmannia [root] (*shēng dì*), which are sweet and cold, to clear the internal heat and nourish the *yīn qì*.

Mulberry Leaf and Chrysanthemum Beverage (*Sāng Jú Yǐn* 桑菊飲)
From the *Detailed Analysis of Warm Diseases* (*Wēn Bìng Tiáo Biàn* 溫病條辯)

apricot kernel (*xìng rén*)	杏仁	6g
forsythia [fruit] (*lián qiào*)	連翹	5g
mulberry leaf (*sāng yè*)	桑葉	8g
chrysanthemum [flower] (*jú huā*)	菊花	3g
platycodon [root] (*kǔ jié gěng*)	苦桔梗	6g
raw licorice [root] (*shēng gān cǎo*)	生甘草	2g
phragmites [root] (*wěi gēn*) (i.e., *lú gēn*)	葦根	6g
mint (*bò hé*) (add later)	薄荷	2g

Give two packets per day. Boil in two cups of water until one cup is left.

Mulberry Leaf and Chrysanthemum Beverage (*Sāng Jú Yǐn*) is an acrid cool exterior-resolving formula, but one that does not have a strong exterior-resolving heat-discharging function. As Wú Jú Tōng remarked, it is a "mild, acrid cooling formula." In it:

- § Mulberry leaf (*sāng yè*), chrysanthemum [flower] (*jú huā*), forsythia [fruit] (*lián qiào*), and mint (*bò hé*), all of which are acrid and cool, mildly outthrust and discharge warm heat.
- § Platycodon [root] (*jié gěng*), licorice [root] (*gān cǎo*), and apricot kernel (*xìng rén*) disinhibit and outthrust lung *qì* to stop coughing.

§ Phragmites [root] (*lú gēn*) engenders fluids and stops thirst.

Both Mulberry Leaf and Chrysanthemum Beverage (*Sāng Jú Yǐn*) and Lonicera and Forsythia Powder (*Yín Qiào Sǎn*) are acrid cool exterior-resolving formulas, suitable for attacks to the lung defense system by wind-heat. The main difference between them is as follows:

Lonicera and Forsythia Powder (*Yín Qiào Sǎn*) contains schizonepeta (*jīng jiè*) and fermented soybean (*dòu chǐ*), both of which are acrid and exterior-resolving. Consequently its exterior-resolving properties are much stronger than those of Mulberry Leaf and Chrysanthemum Beverage (*Sāng Jú Yǐn*).

Mulberry Leaf and Chrysanthemum Beverage (*Sāng Jú Yǐn*) although constituted mainly of acrid cool medicinals, contains them in smaller dosages than Lonicera and Forsythia Powder (*Yín Qiào Sǎn*). It is weaker at resolving the exterior, but because it also contains apricot kernel (*xìng rén*), which downbears lung *qì*, it is stronger at stopping coughs.

Modifications

1. For heat entering the *qì* aspect and causing rough, asthma-like breathing, add gypsum (*shí gāo*) and anemarrhena [root] (*zhī mǔ*) to clear heat from the *qì* aspect.

2. For heat beginning to enter the construction aspect and causing extreme redness of the tongue, dusk-fever, and agitation, add water buffalo horn (*shuǐ niú jiǎo*) and scrophularia [root] (*xuán shēn*) to clear the construction and discharge the heat.

3. For heat entering the blood aspect, replace mint (*bò hé*) and phragmites [root] (*wěi gēn*) with ophiopogon [tuber] (*mài dōng*), raw rehmannia [root] (*shēng dì*), Solomon's seal [root] (*yù zhú*), and moutan [root bark] (*dān pí*). When heat enters the blood aspect external pathogenic *qì* abates, so there is no longer any need to disperse the exterior by using mint (*bò hé*). Also, thirst usually ends so it is no longer necessary to engender fluids and stop thirst by using phragmites [root] (*wěi gēn*). Instead, heat in the blood tends to damage the *yīn* construction, so ophiopogon [tuber] (*mài dōng*), raw rehmannia [root] (*shēng dì*), Solomon's seal [root] (*yù zhú*), and moutan [root bark] (*dān pí*) are needed to cool blood and engender *yīn*.

4. To clear strong lung heat add scutellaria [root] (*huáng qín*).

5. If heat damages the fluids and causes thirst, add trichosanthes root (*tiān huā fěn*) to clear heat and engender fluids.

B. DISEASE PATTERNS AND THEIR TREATMENTS IN HEAT ENTERING THE *QÌ* ASPECT

1. HEAT IN THE CHEST AND DIAPHRAGM

Heat confined in the chest and diaphragm

Pattern

Body heat, vexation, anguish in the heart, agitated movement, and slightly yellow tongue moss.

This pattern occurs when pathogenic *qì*, although already resolved at the exterior, has entered the *qì* aspect at the chest and diaphragm causing body heat, vexation, anguish in the heart, and agitated movement. Even though there is internal pathogenic *qì*, the [pathogenic] heat is not very strong and the fluids have not been damaged, so the fever is usually not very high, the tongue moss is only slightly yellow, the tongue is not dry, and there is absence of thirst.

Treatment

Clear and diffuse the confined heat.

Prescription

Gardenia and Fermented Soybean Decoction (*Zhī Zǐ Chǐ Tāng* 梔子豉湯)

From the *Treatise on Cold Damage* (*Shāng Hán Lùn* 傷寒論)

gardenia [fruit] (*zhī zǐ*)	梔子	10g
unsalted fermented soybean (*dàn dòu chǐ*)	淡豆豉	6g

Boil in water, remove the residue, divide the decoction into two separate doses, and give both doses on the same day.

This formula contains:

- Gardenia [fruit] (*zhī zǐ*), which clears heat.
- Unsalted fermented soybean (*dàn dòu chǐ*), which diffuses confinement and outthrusts the exterior.

The combined effect of these medicinals is to clear and diffuse confined heat from the chest and diaphragm.

Modifications

1. If external pathogens have not been resolved add mint (*bò hé*) and arctium [seed] (*niú bàng zǐ*) to resolve the exterior and outthrust the pathogenic *qì*.

2. If the liquid has been damaged and thirst occurs add trichosanthes root (*tiān huā fěn*) to regenerate the fluids and stop the thirst.

3. If the middle *qì* is insufficient add licorice [root] (*gān cǎo*) to supplement the middle and relax the violent symptoms.

4. If *qì* counterflow causes vomiting add ginger [mix-fried] bamboo shavings (*jiāng zhú rú*) to downbear the counterflow and stop the vomiting.

Heat scorching the chest and diaphragm

Pattern

Incessant body heat, vexation with agitation and disquietude, deflagration-like scorching heat in the chest and diaphragm, charred lips, dry throat, thirst or constipation, red tongue, yellow tongue moss or yellow-white tongue moss with insufficient moisture, and slippery rapid pulse.

These symptoms are caused by pathogenic heat scorching the chest and diaphragm. Pathogenic heat passes from the exterior to the interior, and interior heat becomes exuberant, so body heat is incessant. Heat scorches the chest and diaphragm so vexation, agitation, and disquietude occur with deflagration-like scorching heat in the chest and diaphragm. Heat is exuberant in the upper burner so there is thirst, the lips are charred, and the throat is dry. There is also exuberant heat internally so the tongue moss is yellow or yellow and white with insufficient moisture, and the pulse is slippery and rapid. Constipation results because bowel *qì* is unable to downbear. This is easy to differentiate from a *yáng* brightness bowel repletion heat bind pattern because the abdomen is soft rather than hard, distended, and painful, and the pulse is neither sunken nor replete.

Treatment

Clear and discharge the diaphragm heat.

Prescription

Diaphragm-Cooling Powder (*Liáng Gé Sǎn* 涼膈散)

From the *Imperial Grace Formulary* (*Hé Jì Jú Fāng* 和劑局方).

rhubarb (*dà huáng*) (soaked in alcohol)	大黃	60g
mirabilite (*máng xiāo*)	芒硝	30g
licorice [root] (*gān cǎo*)	甘草	18g
gardenia [fruit] (*zhī zǐ*) (stir baked until brown)	梔子	25g
mint (*bò hé*)	薄荷	20g
scutellaria [root] (*huáng qín*) (stir fried in alcohol)	黃芩	30g
forsythia [fruit] (*lián qiào*)	連翹	30g

Grind all the medicinals into powder. Use 12 or 15g to 30g per dose. Add 15 pieces of bamboo leaf (*zhú yè*) and boil in water. Remove the residue and administer the decoction while still warm. Give three times per day and twice per night. Discontinue treatment when the hot symptoms disappear.

This formula consists of:

- § Forsythia [fruit] (*lián qiào*), mint (*bò hé*), bamboo leaf (*zhú yè*), gardenia [fruit] (*shān zhī zǐ*), and scutellaria [root] (*huáng qín*), which clear and discharge heat pathogens from the chest and diaphragm.
- § Rhubarb (*dà huáng*), mirabilite (*máng xiāo*), and licorice [root] (*gān cǎo*), which throughclear the bowels and conduct heat downward.

The overall effect of these medicinals is to clear heat pathogens from the chest and diaphragm. They can be used as a combination whenever there is heat in the chest and diaphragm and the *yáng* brightness bowel is replete.

Phlegm-heat binding in the chest

Pattern

Red complexion and body heat, unquenchable thirst with desire for cold drinks, vomiting after drinking, dilations and fullness in the chest and stomach duct, constipation, and slippery yellow tongue moss.

These symptoms are caused by pathogenic heat entering the interior and binding with phlegm in the chest and stomach duct. Red complexion and body heat, plus thirst with desire for cold drinks, are caused by exuberant heat at the interior. Phlegm-heat obstructs internally and prevents fluids from rising so thirst is unquenchable and vomiting occurs after drinking. Dilations and fullness in the chest and stomach duct are reflections of phlegm-fire binding in the chest and stomach duct. They are the key symptoms of this pattern and are always accompanied by tenderness. Constipation occurs when internally obstructed pathogens negate the throughclearing function of stomach *qì*; and slippery yellow tongue moss results from phlegm-fire.

The symptoms of red complexion, body heat, and unquenchable thirst with desire for cold drinks make this condition appear similar to *yáng* brightness exuberant heat without form. In this case however the tongue moss is slippery and yellow rather than dry and yellow, and there are also dilations and fullness in the chest and stomach duct—symptoms that are uncharacteristic of *yáng* brightness exuberant heat without form. The symptom of constipation is common to this condition and that of a replete *yáng* brightness bowel disease, but in this case the abdomen is neither distended nor painful, and the tongue moss is not thick, yellow, and dry, as it would be in a repletion bowel disease.

In this and the previous two conditions, the pathogen is in the chest and diaphragm, but in the previous two conditions the pathogenesis and key symptoms are different. In heat confinement in the chest and diaphragm the key symptoms are vexation, agitation, and disquietude, in heat scorching the chest and diaphragm the key symptoms are sensations of scorching heat in the chest and diaphragm and dry throat. Both conditions are caused by pathogenic heat without form, not by turbid phlegm, so in both conditions the tongue moss although yellow is not slippery. This condition, on the other hand, results from phlegm-heat binding in the chest and stomach duct—the key symptoms are dilations and fullness in the chest and stomach duct. Since there is a phlegm-heat bind, the tongue moss must be yellow and slippery or yellow and slimy.

Treatment

Clear the heat, transform the phlegm, and open the binding.

Prescription

Minor Chest Bind Decoction Plus Unripe Bitter Orange
(*Xiǎo Xiàn Xiōng Jiā Zhǐ Shí Tāng* 小陷胸加枳實湯)

From the *Detailed Analysis of Warm Diseases* (*Wēn Bìng Tiáo Biàn* 溫病條辯)

coptis [root] (*huáng lián*)	黃連	6g
trichosanthes [fruit] (*guā lóu*)	栝蔞	10g
unripe bitter orange (*zhǐ shí*)	枳實	6g
pinellia [tuber] (*bàn xià*)	半夏	12g

Boil in five cups of water until two cups are left. Give twice daily.

This prescription consists of Minor Chest Bind Decoction (*Shǎo Xiàn Xiōng Tāng*), which is a *Treatise on Cold Damage* formula, plus unripe bitter orange (*zhǐ shí*). In it:

- Coptis [root] (*huáng lián*) clears heat.
- Trichosanthes [fruit] (*guā lóu*) relaxes the chest and transforms phlegm.
- Pinellia [tuber] (*bàn xià*) transforms phlegm, calms the stomach, and stops vomiting.
- Unripe bitter orange (*zhǐ shí*) downbears *qì* and opens binding.

Its overall function is to clear heat, transform phlegm, and open binding. In the *Treatise on Cold Damage*, Minor Chest Bind Decoction (*Shǎo Xiàn Xiōng Tāng*) was used as a key formula for symptoms of confined phlegm-heat in the chest. Later, to improve its effectiveness, Wú Jú Tōng supplemented it with unripe bitter orange (*zhǐ shí*).

2. PATHOGENIC HEAT IN THE LUNGS

Pathogenic heat congests the lungs

Pattern

Body heat, sweating, vexation and thirst, coughing, dyspnea, oppression in the chest and chest pain, phlegm that is sticky and difficult to expectorate, red tongue, yellow tongue moss, and rapid pulse.

These symptoms usually result when pathogens in the lung defense fail to resolve and successfully develop one more step. Steaming of confined lung heat creates body heat with sweating, so heat damages fluids and there are symptoms of vexation and thirst with increased intake of fluids. Pathogenic heat congests the lungs and prevents lung *qì* from diffusing, so there are also symptoms of coughing, dyspnea, oppression in the chest, chest pain, and sticky phlegm that is difficult to expectorate. The symptoms of yellow tongue moss and rapid pulse both result from internal heat.

Although these symptoms are located in the lungs, they differ from those seen during the initial stages of wind warmth. During the initial stages of wind warmth, besides the expressions of pathogenic *qì* damaging the lung defense, there are also symptoms of aversion to cold and white tongue moss.

Treatment

Clear the heat and diffuse the lung *qì*.

Prescription

Ephedra, Apricot Kernel, Gypsum, and Licorice Decoction
(*Má Xìng Shí Gān Tāng* 麻杏石甘湯)

From the *Treatise on Cold Damage* (*Shāng Hán Lùn* 傷寒論)

ephedra (*má huáng*) (remove the nodes)	麻黃	120g
apricot kernel (*xìng rén*) (remove husk and tips)	杏仁	50pc
honey-fried licorice [root] (*zhì gān cǎo*)	炙甘草	60g
gypsum (*shí gāo*) (crush and wrap in cloth)	石膏	180g

Boil all the medicinals in water and give the decoction while still warm, twice daily.

In this formula:

- Ephedra (*má huáng*) and apricot kernel (*xìng rén*) diffuse lung *qì*.
- Gypsum (*shí gāo*) clears and discharges internal heat.
- Licorice [root] (*gān cǎo*) harmonizes the other ingredients.

Combined, these medicinals clear and diffuse lung heat. Since ephedra (*má huáng*) is acrid and warming, it normally promotes sweating and resolves the exterior; since gypsum (*shí gāo*) is acrid and cold, it is particularly good at clearing *yáng* brightness *qì* aspect heat. But when these two medicinals are used together, the ability of ephedra (*má huáng*) to promote sweating and resolve the exterior diminishes, while its ability to diffuse the lungs and stabilize dyspnea optimizes; the ability of gypsum (*shí gāo*) to clear and discharge *yáng* brightness heat decreases, while its ability to clear and diffuse pathogenic heat from the lungs increases. This prescription has an acrid cool scattering function, so it is used to treat lung heat with external symptoms.

Phlegm-heat obstructing the lungs; heat binding in the bowel

Pattern

Tidal fever and constipation, dyspneic-tachypnea with disquietude, phlegm-drool congestion, big replete right inch pulse, and yellow slimy or yellow slippery tongue moss.

These symptoms occur when the hand greater *yīn* lung and hand *yáng* brightness large intestines are diseased simultaneously. Tidal fever and constipation result from binding of repletion heat in the *yáng* brightness bowel. Dyspneic-tachypnea and big replete right inch pulse result from phlegm-heat obstructing the lungs and preventing the lung *qì* from diffusing and downbearing. And slimy yellow or slippery yellow tongue moss results from internal blockage of phlegm-heat. Since the lung and intestines are internal-external partners, when lung *qì* is unable to downbear it is difficult for bowel *qì* to move, and when heat binds in the intestines there is little chance that the pathogenic heat in the lungs will be able to discharge. It can therefore be seen that this condition results from an interacting of lung and intestine pathogens.

Both these symptoms and the symptoms in the immediately preceding condition are caused by pathogenic heat in the lungs. In both cases there are symptoms of body heat, thirst, coughing, and chest confinement. The difference between them is that in this condition there are also symptoms of phlegm-drool congestion and usually the repletion bowel symptom of constipation.

Treatment

Diffuse the lungs and transform the phlegm, discharge the heat and attack below.

Prescription

White-Diffusing Qì-Infusing Decoction
(*Xuān Bái Chéng Qì Tāng* 宣白承氣湯)

From the *Detailed Analysis of Warm Diseases* (*Wēn Bìng Tiáo Biàn* 溫病條辯)

crude gypsum (*shēng shí gāo*)	生石膏	15g
raw rhubarb (*shēng dà huáng*) (add later)	生大黃	10g
apricot kernel powder (*xìng rén fěn*)	杏仁粉	6g
trichosanthes rind (*guā lóu pí*)	栝蔞皮	5g

Boil in five cups of water until two cups are left. Give one cup and if unsuccessful give the other cup.

When phlegm-heat is trapped in the lung, treatment must be aimed at clearing the lungs and transforming phlegm, and when repletion heat binds in the bowel, treatment must be aimed at attacking below. Therefore, on the one hand, this formula contains apricot kernel (*xìng rén*) and gypsum (*shí gāo*) which clear heat and diffuse lung *qì*, as well as trichosanthes rind (*guā lóu pí*), which clears the lungs and transforms phlegm. By clearing heat and transforming phlegm these medicinals relieve dyspnea. On the other hand, it also contains rhubarb (*dà huáng*), which attacks below to treat bowel repletion.

When bowel repletion is relieved below, lung heat clears easily, and when lung *qì* downbears, bowel *qì* throughclears easily. Together, these medicinals not only clear and diffuse lung heat but also throughclear bowel *qì*. Moreover, by analyzing the actions of its ingredients, it can be seen that this formula adopts the lung *qì* diffusing approach of Ephedra, Apricot Kernel, Gypsum, and Licorice Decoction (*Má Xìng Shí Gān Tāng*), and the bowel *qì* throughclearing approach of Qì-Infusing Decoction (*Chéng Qì Tāng*). It is therefore called White-Diffusing Qì-Infusing Decoction (*Xuān Bái Chéng Qì Tāng*).

Lung heat surfacing as papules

Pattern

Body heat, coughing, oppression in the chest, and red papules on the skin.

These symptoms are caused mostly by lung channel *qì* aspect heat pathogens affecting the construction network vessels. Body heat without aversion to cold occurs because external pathogens enter the lung channel *qì* aspect. Coughing and oppression in the chest occur because heat is confined and lung *qì* is not diffusing. And external papules occur because lung heat affects the construction aspect and moves through the blood network vessels. As Lù Zǐ Xián (陸子賢) explained in his *Six Causes Differentiation* (*Liù Yīn Tiáo Biàn* 六因條辯), "Macules are caused by *yáng* brightness heat toxins, whereas papules are caused by greater *yīn* wind-heat." In wind warmth the core of pathogenic change is in the lung, so when the disease progresses, it can easily lead to surfacing of papules. This is one of the characteristics of this condition.

Treatment

Diffuse the lung and discharge the heat. Cool the construction and outthrust the papules.

Prescription

Lonicera and Forsythia Powder (*Yín Qiào Săn* 銀翹散)

—In which fermented soybean (*dòu chǐ* 豆豉) has been replaced with raw rehmannia [root] (*shēng dì* 生地), moutan [root bark] (*dān pí* 丹皮), isatis leaf (*dà qīng yè* 大青葉), and scrophularia [root] (*xuán shēn* 玄參)—

From the *Detailed Analysis of Warm Diseases* (*Wēn Bìng Tiáo Biàn* 溫病條辯)

lonicera [flower] (*jīn yín huā*)	金銀花	10g
forsythia [fruit] (*lián qiào*)	連翹	10g
platycodon [root] (*jié gěng*)	桔梗	6g
arctium [seed] (*niú bàng zǐ*) (crush)	牛蒡子	10g
mint (*bò hé*) (add later)	薄荷	6g
schizonepeta (*jīng jiè*)	荊芥	12g
bamboo leaf (*dàn zhú yè*)	淡竹葉	10g
fresh phragmites [root] (*xiān lú gēn*)	鮮蘆根	10g
raw licorice [root] (*shēng gān cǎo*)	生甘草	6g
raw rehmannia [root] (*shēng dì*)	生地	12g
isatis leaf (*dà qīng yè*)	大青葉	10g
moutan [root bark] (*dān pí*)	丹皮	10g
scrophularia [root] (*xuán shēn*)	玄參	30g

This formula was originally designed as an acrid cool exterior-resolving prescription for diffusing the lungs and discharging heat, and was originally used to treat patterns caused by pathogenic *qì* attacking the lung defense. But since the pathogen in the above condition is not external, fermented soybean (*dòu chǐ*) has been deleted, and since there are papules that result from lung heat attacking *yīn*, raw rehmannia [root] (*shēng dì*), moutan [root bark] (*dān pí*), isatis leaf (*dà qīng yè*), and scrophularia [root] (*xuán shēn*) have been added to cool *yīn* and scatter toxins. Used together, these medicinals not only diffuse the lungs and discharge heat, but also cool construction and outthrust papules.

3. HEAT IN YÁNG BRIGHTNESS

Exuberant heat without form

Pattern

High fever with great sweating, red complexion, vexation, thirst with desire to drink cold water, dry yellow tongue moss, and big surging or slippery rapid pulse.

These symptoms are caused mostly by exuberant *yáng* brightness interior heat. The pathogen is exuberant and the right [*qì*] is effulgent so the battle between them creates steaming of internal heat and consequently high fever, great sweating, red complexion, and vexation. The pathogen is in the *qì* aspect, not at the exterior, so the high fever is not accompanied by aversion to cold. Steaming of internal heat causes not only red complexion and vexation, but also red eyes. Exuberance of internal heat causes great sweating, (which damages the fluids) and thirst with desire to drink cold water (as a direct response to the fluid damage). The dry yellow tongue moss and the surging big or slippery rapid pulse are both indicative of exuberant internal heat.

Treatment

Clear the heat and engender the liquid.

Prescription

White Tiger Decoction (*Bái Hǔ Tāng* 白虎湯)

From the *Treatise on Cold Damage* (*Shāng Hán Lùn* 傷寒論)

anemarrhena [root] (*zhī mǔ*)	知母	180g
gypsum (*shí gāo*)	石膏	500g
honey-fried licorice [root] (*zhì gān cǎo*)	炙甘草	60g
round-grained nonglutinous rice (*jīng mǐ*)	粳米	6 handfuls

Boil all four medicinals in one deciliter of water. Cook until the round-grained nonglutinous rice (*jīng mǐ*) is ready, then remove the residue and administer the decoction in one-liter doses, while still warm, three times per day.

White Tiger Decoction (*Bái Hǔ Tāng*) can be used whenever exuberant *yáng* brightness *qì* aspect heat damages liquid.

This formula contains:

§ Gypsum (*shí gāo*), which is acrid, cold, internal heat clearing, and discharging.

§ Anemarrhena [root] (*zhī mǔ*), which is bitter, moisturizing, heat clearing, and liquid engendering.

§ Licorice [root] (*gān cǎo*) and round-grained nonglutinous rice (*jīng mǐ*), which are stomach-nourishing and liquid-engendering.

The main action of this combination is to clear heat and safeguard liquid. If this action is not powerful enough, strengthen it by adding medicinals such as lonicera [flower] (*jīn yín huā*), dendrobium [stem] (*shí hú*), and fresh phragmites [root] (*xiān lú gēn*). If fluids have been damaged by exuberant heat, so that there are additional symptoms of aversion to cold in the back and surging big scallion-stalk pulse, add ginseng (*rén shēn*) to clear heat, boost *qì*, and engender liquid.

Binding of heat with form

Pattern

Tidal fevers, episodes of delirious speech, constipation or passing of watery excreta from the bowels, abdominal distention with hardness and pain, dry yellow or dry dark-gray tongue moss, and sunken strong pulse.

These symptoms are caused mostly by pathogenic *qì* in the lung channel, which instead of resolving, enters directly into the stomach and develops into *yáng* brightness bowel repletion. The pathogenic heat has already penetrated deeply, so during the afternoons, when the *yáng* heat (of the body) becomes naturally exuberant, the cyclic intensifying of the battle between right [*qì*] and pathogens creates tidal fevers. Also, the internal heat steams the spirit light (i.e., mind and emotional activities) creating delirious speech, and binds with the stools in the intestines causing constipation, unless the stools with which it binds are dry—in which case nothing but watery excreta is passed from the bowels.

This is known as heat bind circumfluence. In it, the watery excreta smell very foul and are usually accompanied by [painful] burning sensations at the anal sphincter. Regardless of whether there is constipation or heat bind circumfluence, the passage of stools is always blocked by the internal bind, so there is always pain and this is always accompanied by abdominal distention with hardness and tenderness. The remaining symptoms of dry yellow or dry dark-gray tongue moss and sunken strong pulse are both reflections of internal heat bind.

Treatment

Soften the hardness, attack below, and discharge the heat.

Prescription

Stomach-Regulating Qì-Infusing Decoction
(*Tiáo Wèi Chéng Qì Tāng* 調胃承氣湯)
From the *Treatise on Cold Damage* (*Shāng Hán Lùn* 傷寒論)

honey-fried licorice [root] (*zhì gān cǎo*)	炙甘草	60g
mirabilite (*máng xiāo*)	芒硝	250g
rhubarb (*dà huáng*) (Wash with alcohol)	大黃	120g

Boil the licorice [root] (*gān cǎo*) and rhubarb (*dà huáng*) in three liters of water until one liter is left. Remove the residue, then add the mirabilite (*máng xiāo*) and simmer slowly until the water begins to seethe. Administer while still warm.

Intestinal dry bind and repletion heat require that appropriate steps be taken to soften hardness, attack below, and discharge heat. Unless these steps are taken, it not only becomes impossible to eliminate the dry bind, but also to resolve the pathogenic heat. Consequently, Stomach-Regulating Qì-Infusing Decoction (*Tiáo Wèi Chéng Qì Tāng*) is prescribed.

In this formula:

§ Rhubarb (*dà huáng*), which is bitter and cooling, attacks below and discharges heat.

§ Mirabilite (*máng xiāo*), which is salty and cold, softens hardness and moistens dryness.

§ Licorice [root] (*gān cǎo*) moderates the actions of the mirabilite (*máng xiāo*) and rhubarb (*dà huáng*)—it moderates downward evacuation enough for co-action below to resolve the dry bind and confined heat.

If the abdomen is particularly distended, consider adding bitter orange (*zhǐ qiào*) and magnolia bark (*hòu pò*) to move *qì* and break hardness. But bear in mind that since both these medicinals are warming and drying, whenever fluid damage is severe, caution must be exercised. If the moss is dark-black and dry, which is an indication that the bowel has been seriously damaged, add medicinals such as scrophularia [root] (*xuán shēn*), ophiopogon [tuber] (*mài dōng*), and raw rehmannia [root] (*shēng dì*). These three medicinals comprise the formula Humor-Increasing Qì-Infusing Decoction (*Zēng Yè Chéng Qì Tāng*), which attacks below and discharges heat, engenders liquid and nourishes humor.

Intestinal heat diarrhea

Pattern

Body heat, diarrhea, scorching heat at the anus, yellow tongue moss, and rapid pulse.

These symptoms are caused by pathogenic heat in the lungs and stomach shifting down to the large intestines. Pathogenic heat interiorizes so there is body heat that does not abate. The lungs and large intestines are exterior-interior partners. Pathogenic heat hurriedly pours into the large intestines, so there is diarrhea with scorching heat at the anus, and usually yellow watery very foul-smelling stools. Yellow moss and rapid pulse are both reflections of internal heat.

The symptoms of foul-smelling watery excreta and scorching heat at the anus are also seen in heat bind circumfluence. In heat bind circumfluence however, internal binding of dry stools forces watery excreta to pass down the sides of the intestines so that when the bowels move, nothing but foul-smelling water is passed—the abdomen therefore is always tender when pressed. Conversely, in this pattern, the transfer of heat to the intestines usually causes the stools to turn yellow and soft. Since the stools are not dry internally, the abdomen is not sensitive to pressure.

Treatment

Use bitter cold medicinals to clear heat and stop diarrhea.

Prescription

Pueraria, Scutellaria, and Coptis Decoction
(*Gé Gēn Huáng Qín Huáng Lián Tāng* 葛根黃芩黃連湯)
From the *Treatise on Cold Damage* (*Shāng Hán Lùn* 傷寒論)

pueraria [root] (*gé gēn*)	葛根	250g
honey-fried licorice [root] (*zhì gān cǎo*)	炙甘草	60g
scutellaria [root] (*huáng qín*)	黃芩	90g
coptis [root] (*huáng lián*)	黃連	90g

First boil the pueraria [root] (*gé gēn*) in eight liters of water until six liters are left, then add the other ingredients and continue boiling until four liters are left. Remove the residue and administer the decoction while warm.

In this formula:

§ Pueraria [root] (*gé gēn*), which is floating and pure, clears heat and stops diarrhea.

§ Scutellaria [root] (*huáng qín*) and coptis [root] (*huáng lián*), which are bitter and cold, directly clear internal heat.

§ Licorice [root] (*gān cǎo*), which is sweet, relaxes the center.

Once the intestinal heat clears the diarrhea stops. For vomiting, add agastache (*huò xiāng*) and ginger [mix-fried] bamboo shavings (*jiāng zhú rú*). For abdominal pain add white peony [root] (*bái sháo*).

C. DISEASE PATTERNS AND THEIR TREATMENTS IN HEAT TRAPPED AT THE PERICARDIUM

1. COUNTERFLOW INTO THE PERICARDIUM

Pattern

Scorching body heat, clouding of the spirit with delirious speech or coma without speech, sluggish tongue, and limb reversal.

These symptoms are caused mainly by pathogens passing from the lung defense into the pericardium. As Yè Tiān Shì indicated, "Pathogenic warmth enters from above, attacks the lungs first and then counterflows into the pericardium." Pathogenic heat falls internally, the fluids are scorched into phlegm, phlegm-heat blocks and obstructs the pericardium network vessels, and the spirit mind [i.e., conscious mind] is disturbed. Consequently, there is clouding of the spirit with delirious speech, or coma without speech. The tongue is the "sprout" of the heart. Phlegm-heat blocks the heart orifices, so the tongue becomes sluggish and the person's speech becomes slurred. Pathogenic heat obstructs internally, so the body steams with scorching heat while the arms and legs suffer reversal cold. If heat is obstructed shallowly, the limb reversal is only mildly cold, but if heat is obstructed more deeply, their reversal is severe—in other words, "when heat is deep, reversal is also deep; when heat is mild, reversal is also mild."

Treatment

Clear the heart and open the orifices.

Prescription

Palace-Clearing Decoction (*Qīng Gōng Tāng* 清宮湯) given with Peaceful Palace Bovine Bezoar Pill (*Ān Gōng Niú Huáng Wán* 安宮牛黃丸) or Purple Snow Elixir (*Zǐ Xuě Dān* 紫雪丹) or Supreme Jewel Elixir (*Zhì Bǎo Dān* 至寶丹).

Palace-Clearing Decoction (*Qīng Gōng Tāng* 清宮湯)

From the *Detailed Analysis of Warm Diseases* (*Wēn Bìng Tiáo Biàn* 溫病條辯)

tender scrophularia [root] (*xuán shēn xīn*)	玄參心	10g
lotus embryo (*lián zǐ xīn*)	連子心	2g
tender bamboo leaf (*zhú yè xīn*)	竹葉心	6g
tender forsythia [fruit] (*lián qiào xīn*)	連翹心	6g
rhinoceros horn tip (*xī jiǎo jiān*)	犀角尖	6g
[mix-fried] ophiopogon [tuber] (*lián xīn mài dōng*)	連心麥冬	10g

These days, use 18g of water buffalo horn (*shuǐ niú jiǎo*) instead of 6g of rhinoceros horn tip (*xī jiǎo jiān*).

Peaceful Palace Bovine Bezoar Pill
(*Ān Gōng Niú Huáng Wán* 安宮牛黃丸)

From the *Detailed Analysis of Warm Diseases* (*Wēn Bìng Tiáo Biàn* 溫病條辯)

bovine bezoar (*niú huáng*)	牛黃	30g
curcuma [tuber] (*yù jīn*)	鬱金	30g
rhinoceros horn (*xī jiǎo*)	犀角	30g
coptis [root] (*huáng lián*)	黃連	30g
cinnabar (*zhū shā*)	朱砂	30g
borneol (*bīng piàn*)	冰片	7g
musk (*shè xiāng*)	麝香	7g
pearl (*zhēn zhū*)	珍珠	15g
gardenia [fruit] (*shān zhī*)	山梔	30g
realgar (*xióng huáng*)	雄黃	30g
scutellaria [root] (*huáng qín*)	黃芩	30g

These days, use 90g of water buffalo horn (*shuǐ niú jiǎo*) instead of 30g of rhinoceros horn (*xī jiǎo*). Grind all the ingredients into powder; combine with honey and press into three-gram pills. Then cover with goldleaf and protect with wax. If the pulse is vacuous administer this prescription with Ginseng Decoction (*Rén Shēn Tāng*); if replete, with Lonicera [flower] and Mint Decoction (*Yín Huā Bò Hé Tāng*). For pestilence diseases like "flying body sudden syncope" and "five convulsions penetrating fear," in which patients suffer from hot type tetanic reversals, give one pill per dose. Constitutionally strong adult patients should be given two or three doses per day, but infants should be given only half a pill, and then, if this does not produce the desired results, another half a pill.

Purple Snow Elixir (*Zǐ Xuě Dān* 紫雪丹)

From the *Detailed Analysis of Warm Diseases* (*Wēn Bìng Tiáo Biàn* 溫病條辯)

talcum (*huá shí*)	滑石	500g
gypsum (*shí gāo*)	石膏	500g
glauberite (*hán shuǐ shí*)	寒水石	500g
loadstone (*cí shí*)	磁石	1000g
antelope horn (*líng yáng jiǎo*)	羚羊角	150g
saussurea [root] (*mù xiāng*)	木香	150g
rhinoceros horn (*xī jiǎo*)	犀角	150g
aquilaria [wood] (*chén xiāng*)	沉香	150g
clove (*dīng xiāng*)	丁香	30g
cimicifuga [root] (*shēng má*)	升麻	30g
scrophularia [root] (*xuán shēn*)	玄參	500g
honey-fried licorice [root] (*zhì gān cǎo*)	炙甘草	240g

These days, use 450g of water buffalo horn (*shuǐ niú jiǎo*) instead of 150g of rhinoceros horn (*xī jiǎo*). Grind the first four medicinals, boil them in water, discard the residue and set the decoction aside. Then grind the remaining eight medicinals and boil them in the already prepared decoction. After boiling, remove the residue and set it aside. Next, add 1,000g of impure mirabilite (*pò xiāo*) and 1,000g of niter (*xiāo shí*) to the decoction, steep as a tea, and discard the residue. Following this, add the previously set aside residue and gently simmer while stirring with a weeping willow stick. When it dissolves and the decoction becomes toffee-like, stir in 90g of ground cinnabar (*chén shā*) and 36g of ground musk (*shè xiāng*). Do not stop simmering until they have been thoroughly mixed in. Give three to six grams per dose with cold water.

Imperial Grace Supreme Jewel Elixir (*Jú Fāng Zhì Bǎo Dān* 局方至寶丹)

From the *Detailed Analysis of Warm Diseases* (*Wēn Bìng Tiáo Biàn* 溫病條辯)

rhinoceros horn (*xī jiǎo*) (crushed)	犀角	30g
cinnabar (*zhū shā*) (water-ground)	朱砂	30g
amber (*hǔ pò*) (ground)	琥珀	30g
hawksbill [turtle] shell (*dài mào*) (crushed)	玳瑁	30g
bovine bezoar (*niú huáng*)	牛黄	12g
musk (*shè xiāng*)	麝香	15g

These days, use 30g of water buffalo horn (*shuǐ niú jiǎo*) instead of 10g of rhinoceros horn (*xī jiǎo*). Stew all the ingredients with benzoin (*ān xī xiāng*), make the mixture into about one hundred pills, and protect the pills by coating them in wax.

Palace-Clearing Decoction (*Qīng Gōng Tāng*) is particularly good at clearing pathogenic heat from the pericardium network vessels. Its name is taken from the fact that the pericardium network vessels are sometimes called the palace wall of the heart—palace-clearing means clearing heat from the pericardium. In it:

§ Water buffalo horn (*shuǐ niú jiǎo*) clears heart heat.

§ Tender scrophularia [root] (*xuán shēn xīn*), lotus embryo (*lián zǐ xīn*), and [mix-fried] ophiopogon [tuber] (*lián xīn mài dōng*) clear the heart and moisten humor.

§ Tender bamboo leaf (*zhú yè xīn*) and tender forsythia [fruit] (*lián qiào xīn*) discharge heat.

The overall effect of these medicinals is to resolve pathogenic *qì* from the pericardium. For hot phlegm add dried bamboo sap (*zhú lì*) and trichosanthes rind (*guā lóu pí*), and for closed orifices add acorus [root] (*shí chāng pú*). Traditionally, for particularly strong heat toxins, purified feces (*jīn zhī* or *fèn qīng*), a fluid made by aging human feces, was added. But this medicinal is no longer in clinical use.

Peaceful Palace Bovine Bezoar Pill (*Ān Gōng Niú Huáng Wán*), Purple Snow Elixir (*Zǐ Xuě Dān*), and Supreme Jewel Elixir (*Zhì Bǎo Dān*) are all prepared medicines that clear the heart and open the orifices to revive the spirit mind [i.e., the conscious mind]—but they are all different. Peaceful Palace Bovine Bezoar Pill (*Ān Gōng Niú Huáng Wán*) is better at clearing heat and eliminating toxins, Purple Snow Elixir (*Zǐ Xuě Dān*) is better at extinguishing wind, and Supreme Jewel Elixir (*Zhì Bǎo Dān*) is better at fragrantly opening impurities.

2. HEAT ENTERING THE PERICARDIUM WITH SIMULTANEOUS BOWEL REPLETION

Pattern

Body heat, loss of consciousness, sluggish tongue, limb reversal, constipation, abdominal hardness and tenderness, and unquenchable thirst.

These symptoms are hand reverting *yīn* pericardium and hand *yáng* brightness large intestine symptoms. Since the pericardium is being invaded, body heat, loss of consciousness, sluggish tongue, and limb reversal occur. Since dry stools are trapped in the intestines, constipation with abdominal hardness and tenderness occurs. And since the *yīn* fluids have been damaged by heat, unquenchable thirst also occurs. Of these symptoms, body heat, loss of consciousness, and limb reversal can all occur when the *yáng* brightness bowel is replete, but sluggish tongue, which makes speaking impossible, can only occur when heat has entered the pericardium. This then, is the key symptom.

Treatment

Clear the heart and open the orifices, while simultaneously attacking the bowel repletion below.

Prescription

Bovine Bezoar Qì-Infusing Decoction
(*Niú Huáng Chéng Qì Tāng* 牛黃承氣湯)

From the *Detailed Analysis of Warm Diseases* (*Wēn Bìng Tiáo Biàn* 溫病條辯)

Peaceful Palace Bovine Bezoar Pill (*Ān Gōng Niú Huáng Wán*)	安宮牛黃丸	2 pills
raw rhubarb powder (*shēng dà huáng sǎn*)	生大黃散	10g

Dissolve two Peaceful Palace Bovine Bezoar Pills (*Ān Gōng Niú Huáng Wán*) in warm water, add 10g of raw rhubarb powder (*shēng dà huáng sǎn*) and divide into two portions. If the first portion fails to achieve the desired therapeutic results, give the second.

In this prescription, Peaceful Palace Bovine Bezoar Pill (*Ān Gōng Niú Huáng Wán*) clears heat from the pericardium, and raw rhubarb powder (*shēng dà huáng sǎn*) drains down *yáng* brightness bowel repletion heat. For binding of dryness with more severely damaged fluid, add mirabilite (*máng xiāo*) and scrophularia [root] (*xuán shēn*), which soften and resolve hard lumps and engender fluids. For more severe damage to the pericardium system without severe binding of dryness in the bowels, aim firstly to clear the heart and open the orifices, and then later to attack below.

D. THE DISEASE PATTERN AND ITS TREATMENT IN RESIDUAL UNRESOLVED HEAT DAMAGING THE LUNG AND STOMACH YĪN

Pattern

There may be low fever or not, dry coughing or coughing up small quantities of sticky phlegm, dry mouth and tongue, and thirst.

When these symptoms occur, they are usually seen during the recovery stage of a wind warmth disease. Whether there is retention of residual pathogenic heat with lingering low fever or not, there is always damaged lung and stomach *yīn*. Since the lung fluids have been damaged there is dry coughing or coughing up small quantities of sticky phlegm, and since the stomach fluids have been damaged there is dry mouth and tongue with thirst.

Treatment

Nourish the lung and stomach *yīn* fluids.

Prescription

Adenophora/Glehnia and Ophiopogon Decoction
(*Shā Shēn Mài Mén Dōng Tāng* 沙參麥門冬湯)
From the *Detailed Analysis of Warm Diseases* (*Wēn Bìng Tiáo Biàn* 溫病條辯)

adenophora/glehnia [root] (*shā shēn*)	沙參	10g
Solomon's seal [root] (*yù zhú*)	玉竹	6g
raw licorice [root] (*shēng gān cǎo*)	生甘草	3g
frostbitten mulberry leaf (*dōng sāng yè*)	冬桑葉	5g
ophiopogon [tuber] (*mài dōng*)	麥冬	10g
raw lablab [bean] (*shēng biǎn dòu*)	生扁豆	5g
trichosanthes root (*huā fěn*)	花粉	5g

Boil all seven ingredients in five cups of water and simmer until two cups are left. Give two doses per day, boiling the same packet of medicinals on both occasions.

In this prescription:

- Adenophora/glehnia [root] (*shā shēn*), ophiopogon [tuber] (*mài dōng*), trichosanthes root (*huā fěn*), and Solomon's seal [root] (*yù zhú*) nourish the lung and stomach fluids.
- Lablab [bean] (*biǎn dòu*) and licorice [root] (*gān cǎo*) nourish the stomach *qì*.
- Frostbitten mulberry leaf (*dōng sāng yè*) clears any residual pathogenic heat.

The overall effect of these seven medicinals is to moisten the lung, stop coughing, discharge heat, and soothe the stomach.

CHAPTER 8
SPRING WARMTH

Spring warmth is an acute hot disease caused by spring-season warm heat pathogens, and characterized by internal heat. Its initial symptoms include high fever, unquenchable thirst, and sometimes even clouded spirit and tetanic reversion. Outbreaks usually occur during spring, or within the change between winter and spring. Onsets are normally sudden, conditions serious, and symptoms relatively unstable. Based on their seasonal natures and clinical expressions, wind warmth theory can be applied in pattern differentiation and treatment identification of biomedically defined conditions such as serious influenza and epidemic cerebrospinal meningitis.

I. DISEASE CAUSES AND PATHOLOGY

Spring warmth usually takes form when spring season warm heat pathogens attack people with premature depletions of *yīn* essence and insufficiencies of right *qì*. When right *qì* is insufficient and pathogens assail, they are easily able to enter the interior, so even though the disease is only at its initial stage, its symptoms reflect intensifying of internal heat. Any accompanying external symptoms, such as aversion to cold and headache, disappear very quickly. Since the characteristic symptoms of this disease are very different from the lung defense symptoms that normally occur during the initial stages of most other warm diseases, our predecessors applied the idea that latent cold transforms into warmth (i.e., that "damage by cold during winter must manifest as warm disease during spring"), and classified it a latent *qì* warm disease.

When the only symptoms that occur during the initial stage of this disease are symptoms of internal heat, its outbreaks are called "latent pathogen spontaneous eruptions," but when accompanying external symptoms occur, its outbreaks are called "newly contracted (pathogen) precipitated eruptions." Depending on the severity of the newly contracted pathogen and the extent of right *qì* vacuity, the symptoms of internal heat can erupt in the *qì* or construction aspect. When the pathogen is in the *qì* aspect, even though pathogenic *qì* is exuberant, the ability of right *qì* to resist remains strong, so the disease state is relatively less severe than when the pathogen is in the construction aspect.

If the disease develops, the pathogen can enter the construction or blood aspect. When it enters the construction aspect the pathogenic heat is deeper, and if it depletes *yīn* construction, the disease state is relatively more severe than when the pathogen is in the *qì* aspect. If the disease state changes for the better its focus transfers to the *qì* aspect; if it changes for the worse it transfers to the blood aspect. During the course of this disease (i.e., at the heat-abundant stage), intensifying of internal heat can easily damage the *yīn* fluids or exuberant heat can stir wind. And by the final stage, the heat can have easily damaged the liver and kidney *yīn*, so at this time, when pathogen strength weakens, vacuity can become more prominent.

II. MAIN POINTS OF DIAGNOSIS

1. Externally precipitated hot diseases can be diagnosed as spring warmth when they occur during spring, or within the change between winter and spring, and are characterized by clinical symptoms of high fever, vexation, thirst, and sweating that fails to resolve pathogens. Occasionally, aversion to cold and absence of sweating or scant sweating occurs, but never for long. The external symptoms quickly disappear, leaving only the symptoms of internal heat.

2. During its onset, this condition must be distinguished from wind warmth. For more details see Chapter One.

3. As the disease progresses, papules and macules can easily appear with clouded spirit and tetanic reversion.

III. PATTERN IDENTIFICATION AND TREATMENT DETERMINATION

The main principle for treating this disease is to clear and discharge the internal heat while simultaneously protecting the *yīn* fluids and outthrusting the pathogens. When heat first enters the *qì* aspect, use bitter cold medicinals to directly clear it from the interior. When it enters the construction aspect, aim mainly to clear the construction and resolve the toxins, outthrust the heat and outpush it to the exterior. When there are concurrent external symptoms, clear the internal heat, while simultaneously resolving the external pathogens. When exuberant heat stirs the blood, creating rashes or causing bleeding, clear the heat, cool the blood, and resolve the toxins. When exuberant heat stirs wind, cool the liver and extinguish the wind; and when heat damages the liver and kidney *yīn*, enrich and nourish them.

A. DISEASE PATTERNS AND THEIR TREATMENTS DURING THE INITIAL STAGE

1. ERUPTION [OF SYMPTOMS] IN THE *QÌ* ASPECT PATTERN

Pattern

Fever, bitter taste in the mouth, thirst, vexation, scant yellow urine, red tongue, yellow tongue moss, and string-like rapid pulse.

These are the symptoms characteristically seen during the initial stage of spring warmth, when the pathogen is in the *qì* aspect. Internal pathogenic heat causes fever without aversion to cold. Heat confined to the interior damages fluids, causing vexation, bitter taste in the mouth, and thirst. Scant yellow urine, red tongue, yellow tongue moss, and string-like rapid pulse are all indications of internal heat. Since this disease is marked by symptoms of bitter taste in the mouth, vexation, and string-like pulse, our predecessors considered it a manifestation of heat in the lesser *yáng* gallbladder channel.

In the event of a concurrent external pathogen, besides the above symptoms there will also be headache and aversion to cold with absence of sweating or scant sweating. This is easily distinguishable from wind warmth, during the initial stage of which there are always prominent lung defense symptoms, with few internal heat symptoms.

Treatment

The primary treatment is to directly clear the internal heat with bitter cold medicinals, and when there are concurrent external symptoms, the secondary treatment is to outthrust the exterior.

Prescription

Scutellaria Decoction (*Huáng Qín Tāng* 黃芩湯)
From the *Treatise on Cold Damage* (*Shāng Hán Lùn* 傷寒論)

scutellaria [root] (*huáng qín*)	黃芩	90g
white peony [root] (*bái sháo*)	芍藥	60g
honey-fried licorice [root] (*zhì gān cǎo*)	炙甘草	60g
jujube (*dà zǎo*)	大棗	12pc

Boil all four ingredients in two liters of water until 600 milliliters are left. Remove the residue and give the decoction thrice daily (once in the morning, once at midday, and once at night), in two hundred milliliter doses.

This formula is bitter cold, heat-clearing, and *yīn*-hardening. In it:

§ Scutellaria [root] (*huáng qín*), which is bitter and cold, directly clears internal heat;

§ White peony [root] (*bái sháo*) and licorice [root] (*zhì gān cǎo*), which are sour and sweet, transform *yīn* and engender fluids.

The fact that these medicinals are used at the beginning of a spring warmth disease illustrates that when the principal symptoms are of internal heat damaging *yīn,* the principal treatment should be to clear the heat and harden the *yīn*. In practice however, the prescription must be modified according to the clinical manifestations. Honey-fried licorice [root] (*zhì gān cǎo*), which is warming and reinforcing, should be replaced with raw licorice [root] (*shēng gān cǎo*), which is better at clearing heat and resolving toxins. Jujube (*dà zǎo*), which is warming and reinforcing, should be deleted altogether.

On the other hand, since the aim of treatment is to facilitate the outthrust of pathogenic heat to the exterior and to ensure that fluids are engendered, medicinals such as fermented soybean (*dòu chǐ*) and scrophularia [root] (*xuán shēn*) should be added to strengthen results. Moreover, for concurrent external symptoms, medicinals such as pueraria [root] (*gé gēn*), fermented soybean (*dòu chǐ*), and mint (*bò hé*) should be added to outthrust and resolve.

2. ERUPTION [OF SYMPTOMS] IN THE CONSTRUCTION ASPECT

Pattern

Fever that gets stronger at night, vexation, agitated movement, sometimes delirious speech, dry throat, slight thirst, crimson-red tongue without moss, and fine rapid pulse.

This pattern is usually seen when severe pathogens attack people who have pre-existing construction *yīn* vacuity. So even though spring warmth is still at its initial stage, there are symptoms of heat detriment in the construction *yīn*, and heart spirit harassment. Pathogenic heat detriments the *yīn* construction, so there is fever that gets stronger at night, dry throat, and fine rapid pulse. Construction heat steams upward, so there is crimson-red tongue without moss, and slight thirst. Pathogenic heat enters the construction and construction *qì* throughclears to the heart, so the heart spirit is harassed and there is vexation, agitated movement, and sometimes delirious speech. These symptoms are similar to those of a repletion *yáng* brightness bowel exuberant heat disease with clouded spirit and delirious speech. But there are three important differences—the stools are not tightly bound, the abdomen is not hard and painful, and the tongue moss is not grimy.

If at the same time as a spring warmth pathogen erupts in the construction aspect, an exogenous pathogen attacks the exterior, there will be accompanying symptoms of fever with aversion to cold and headache without sweating or with scant sweating.

Treatment

Clear the construction and discharge the heat. Construction-Clearing Decoction (*Qīng Yíng Tāng*) can be used. If there are accompanying external symptoms, external-outthrusting methods can be used to assist.

Prescription

Construction-Clearing Decoction (*Qīng Yíng Tāng* 清營湯)

From the *Detailed Analysis of Warm Diseases* (*Wēn Bìng Tiáo Biàn* 溫病條辯)

rhinoceros horn (*xī jiǎo*)	犀角	10g
raw rehmannia [root] (*shēng dì*)	生地	15g
scrophularia [root] (*xuán shēn*)	玄參	15g
tender bamboo leaf (*zhú yè xīn*)	竹葉心	3g
ophiopogon [tuber] (*mài dōng*)	麥冬	10g
salvia [root] (*dān shēn*)	丹參	6g
coptis [root] (*huáng lián*)	黃連	5g
lonicera [flower] (*jīn yín huā*)	金銀花	10g
forsythia [fruit] (*lián qiào*) (uncored)	連翹	6g

These days, use 30g of water buffalo horn (*shuǐ niú jiǎo*) instead of 10g of rhinoceros horn (*xī jiǎo*). Boil all the ingredients in eight cups of water until three cups are left. Give in one cup doses three times daily.

In Construction-Clearing Decoction (*Qīng Yíng Tāng* 清營湯):

§ Water buffalo horn (*shuǐ niú jiǎo*) and coptis [root] (*huáng lián*) clear heat from the heart construction.

§ Raw rehmannia [root] (*shēng dì*), scrophularia [root] (*xuán shēn*), ophiopogon [tuber] (*mài dōng*) and salvia [root] (*dān shēn*) clear construction heat and enrich construction *yīn*.

§ Lonicera [flower] (*jīn yín huā*), forsythia [fruit] (*lián qiào*), and bamboo leaf (*zhú yè*), which are floating, diffusing, and heat-discharging, resolve pathogenic heat by shifting it from the construction aspect to the *qì* aspect.

As Yè Tiān Shì said, "[When pathogens] enter the construction [aspect] heat can be outthrust by shifting it to the *qì* [aspect]." If there are accompanying external symptoms, consider adding medicinals such as fermented soybean (*dòu chǐ*), mint (*bò hé*), and arctium [seed] (*niú bàng zǐ*) to diffuse and outthrust the external pathogen.

B. DISEASE PATTERNS AND THEIR TREATMENTS IN BINDING OF HEAT IN THE INTESTINAL BOWEL

1. BOWEL REPLETION WITH CONCURRENT YĪN HUMOR DEPLETION DETRIMENT

Pattern

Fever, abdominal fullness, constipation, dry mouth, cracked lips, and charred dry tongue moss.

Warm pathogens can easily damage *yīn*, so warm diseases with *yáng* brightness bowel repletion are generally accompanied by *yīn* fluid depletion detriment. Internal binding of *yáng* brightness bowel repletion causes fever, abdominal fullness, and constipation; depletion detriment of *yīn* fluids causes dry mouth, cracked lips, and charred dry tongue moss.

Treatment

Enrich the *yīn* and attack below. Humor-Increasing Qì-Infusing Decoction (*Zēng Yè Chéng Qì Tāng*) can be used. After pathogenic heat has been eliminated, if *yīn* humor depletion detriment continues to dry the intestines so that there is still constipation, Humor-Increasing Decoction (*Zēng Yè Tāng*) can be used to enrich the *yīn* and moisten the dryness.

Prescription

Humor-Increasing Qì-Infusing Decoction
(*Zēng Yè Chéng Qì Tāng* 增液承氣湯)
From the *Detailed Analysis of Warm Diseases* (*Wēn Bìng Tiáo Biàn* 溫病條辯)

scrophularia [root] (*xuán shēn*)	玄參	30g
ophiopogon [tuber] (*mài dōng*) (including the core)	麥冬	25g
raw rehmannia [root] (*shēng dì*)	生地	25g
rhubarb (*dà huáng*)	大黃	10g
mirabilite (*máng xiāo*)	芒硝	5g

Boil in five cups of water until three cups are left, wait until it cools and then give one cup. If good results are not forthcoming (after about four to eight hours), give another cup.

This prescription is made by supplementing Humor-Increasing Decoction (*Zēng Yè Tāng*) with mirabilite (*máng xiāo*) and rhubarb (*dà huáng*).

It consists of:

- Scrophularia [root] (*xuán shēn*), raw rehmannia [root] (*shēng dì*), and ophiopogon [tuber] (*mài dōng*) which enrich and nourish *yīn* humor, moisten the intestines, and throughclear the stools.
- Rhubarb (*dà huáng*) and mirabilite (*máng xiāo*) which drain heat, soften hardness, and attack bowel repletion.

These medicinals form a particularly good combination for enriching the *yīn* and attacking below.

Humor-Increasing Decoction (*Zēng Yè Tāng* 增液湯)

From the *Detailed Analysis of Warm Diseases* (*Wēn Bìng Tiáo Biàn* 溫病條辯)

scrophularia [root] (*xuán shēn*)	玄參	30g
ophiopogon [tuber] (*mài dōng*) (including the core)	麥冬	25g
raw rehmannia [root] (*shēng dì*)	生地	25g

Boil in eight cups of water until three cups are left. If there is thirst (dry mouth), give all three cups together. If good results are not forthcoming (if the thirst fails to diminish after about four hours), give another dose.

This prescription consists of liquid-engendering humor-nourishing medicinals, and is therefore called Humor-Increasing Decoction (*Zēng Yè Tāng*). It can only be used when wind warmth disease bowel repletion pathogens have already been eliminated, but dryness of fluids still prevents stools from throughclearing. According to the founding fathers of Chinese medicine, it works by "increasing the water to float the boat."

2. BOWEL REPLETION WITH CONCURRENT VACUITY OF BOTH QÌ AND HUMOR

Pattern

Fever, abdominal fullness, constipation, dry mouth and throat, lassitude of the spirit, fatigue and shortness of breath, yellow or charred-black tongue moss, and sunken weak or sunken rough pulse.

These are symptoms of *yáng* brightness bowel repletion with concurrent vacuity of right *qì*. Fever, abdominal fullness, constipation, and yellow or charred-black tongue moss are the characteristics of a *yáng* brightness bowel repletion pattern. Dry mouth and throat are the characteristics of a *yīn* humor depletion detriment pattern. Lassitude of the spirit, shortness of breath, and sunken weak or sunken rough pulse are characteristics of insufficient right *qì*.

The symptoms of this pattern and those of bowel repletion with concurrent *yīn* humor depletion detriment are both similar in that they both reflect a mixture of vacuity and repletion. But in bowel repletion with concurrent *yīn* humor depletion detriment, the bowel is replete while the *yīn* humor is deplete, whereas in bowel repletion with concurrent vacuity of both *qì* and humor, the bowel is replete while the *qì* and humor are deplete.

Treatment

Attack the bowel repletion below while simultaneously supplementing and boosting the *qì* and humor.

Prescription

Newly Supplemented Yellow Dragon Decoction
(*Xīn Jiā Huáng Lóng Tāng* 新加黄龍湯)
From the *Detailed Analysis of Warm Diseases* (*Wēn Bìng Tiáo Biàn* 溫病條辯)

raw rehmannia [root] (*shēng dì*)	生地	15g
ophiopogon [tuber] (*mài dōng*) (including the core)	麥冬	15g
scrophularia [root] (*xuán shēn*)	玄參	15g
raw rhubarb (*shēng dà huáng*)	生大黃	10g
mirabilite (*máng xiāo*)	芒硝	3g
raw licorice [root] (*shēng gān cǎo*)	生甘草	6g
ginseng (*rén shēn*) (cooked separately)	人參	5g
tangkuei (*dāng guī*)	當歸	5g
sea cucumber (*hǎi shēn*) (washed)	海參	2
ginger juice (*jiāng zhī*)	姜汁	6 spoons

Boil the ingredients in eight cups of water until three cups are left. Initially, give one cup with 3g of the ginseng (*rén shēn*) preparation. Discontinue medication as soon as stools are passed.

This formula is Táo Jié Ān's (陶節庵) Yellow Dragon Decoction (*Huáng Lóng Tāng*). In it:

- § Ginseng (*rén shēn*) and licorice [root] (*gān cǎo*) supplement right *qì*.
- § Rhubarb (*dà huáng*) and mirabilite (*máng xiāo*) drain heat and soften hardness.
- § Ophiopogon [tuber] (*mài dōng*), raw rehmannia [root] (*shēng dì*), scrophularia [root] (*xuán shēn*), and tangkuei (*dāng guī*) enrich *yīn* and moisten dryness.

§ Sea cucumber (*hăi shēn*) enriches and supplements *yīn* humor and softens hardness.

§ Ginger juice (*jiāng zhī*) diffuses and throughclears *qì* aspect binding and stagnation.

When these medicinals are used together, they attack and supplement simultaneously.

3. YÁNG BRIGHTNESS BOWEL REPLETION WITH EXUBERANT SMALL INTESTINE HEAT

Pattern

Fever, constipation, dribbling of urine with inhibited flow and urethral pain, red urine (discolored by bleeding), and sometimes vexation and thirst.

These are symptoms of *yáng* brightness bowel repletion with exuberant small intestine heat. Heat is exuberant at the interior and there is bowel repletion internal blockage, so there is fever and the stools are unable to throughclear. Small intestine heat is exuberant, and it invades the bladder below, so there is dribbling of urine with inhibited flow, urethral pain, and red discoloration. Heat is exuberant and fluids are unable to infuse above so there is vexation and thirst.

Treatment

Throughclear the large intestine blockage and discharge the small intestine heat.

Prescription

Red-Abducting Qì-Infusing Decoction
(*Dăo Chì Chéng Qì Tāng* 導赤承氣湯)
From the *Detailed Analysis of Warm Diseases* (*Wēn Bìng Tiáo Biàn* 溫病條辯)

red peony [root] (*chì sháo*)	赤芍	10g
raw rehmannia [root] (*shēng dì*)	生地	15g
raw rhubarb (*shēng dà huáng*)	生大黃	10g
coptis [root] (*huáng lián*)	黃連	6g
phellodendron [bark] (*huáng băi*)	黃柏	6g
mirabilite (*máng xiāo*)	芒硝	3g

Boil the ingredients in five cups of water until two cups are left. To begin, give one cup, then if no results are forthcoming, after about four hours give another cup.

The reason that this formula is called Red-Abducting *Qì*-Infusing Decoction (*Dǎo Chì Chéng Qì Tāng*) is that it is composed of a modified combination of Red-Abducting Decoction (*Dǎo Chì Tāng*) and Stomach-Regulating *Qì*-Infusing Decoction (*Tiáo Wèi Chéng Qì Tāng*). It contains:

§ Rhubarb (*dà huáng*) and mirabilite (*máng xiāo*), which attack bowel repletion;

§ Raw rehmannia [root] (*shēng dì*), red peony [root] (*chì sháo*), coptis [root] (*huáng lián*), and phellodendron [bark] (*huáng bǎi*), which nourish *yīn* and discharge heat.

C. DISEASE PATTERNS AND THEIR TREATMENTS IN HEAT IN THE CONSTRUCTION-BLOOD ASPECT

1. INTENSE HEAT STIRRING BLOOD

Pattern

Scorching hot body [i.e., high fever], agitation or clouding with mania and delirious raving, dark purple-black rashes or vomiting of blood or nose bleeding or blood in the stools, and dark-crimson tongue.

These are symptoms of intense heat stirring blood. The heart governs the blood and the spirit light. Heat harasses the heart spirit, so there is agitation or clouding with mania and delirious raving. Heat sears the *yīn* blood, so the body is scorching hot. Exuberant heat stirs the blood, so rashes, vomiting of blood, nose bleeding, or blood in the stools can be seen. The rashes are purple-black in color and the tongue is dark-crimson. These symptoms are characteristic of heat toxins deep in the blood aspect.

Treatment

Clear the heat, cool the blood, and resolve the toxins.

Prescription

Rhinoceros Horn and Rehmannia Decoction
(*Xī Jiǎo Dì Huáng Tāng* 犀角地黄湯)

From the *Detailed Analysis of Warm Diseases* (*Wēn Bìng Tiáo Biàn* 溫病條辯)

dried rehmannia [root] (*gān dì huáng*)	干地黄	30g
raw white peony [root] (*shēng bái sháo*)	生白芍	10g
moutan [root bark] (*dān pí*)	丹皮	10g
rhinoceros horn (*xī jiǎo*)	犀角	10g

These days, use 30g of water buffalo horn (*shuǐ niú jiǎo*) instead of 10g of rhinoceros horn (*xī jiǎo*). Boil the ingredients in five cups of water until two cups are left. Give twice daily. Keep the remnants and use them a second time.

This formula consists of:

- Water buffalo horn (*shuǐ niú jiǎo*), which clears heat and resolves toxins.
- Moutan [root bark] (*dān pí*), raw rehmannia [root] (*shēng dì*), and raw white peony [root] (*shēng bái sháo*), which cool and quicken blood.

The overall effect of these medicinals is to clear heat and resolve toxins, and cool and to scatter blood.

2. *QÌ* AND CONSTRUCTION [BLOOD] BOTH SEARED

Pattern

Vigorous fever, thirst, headache, agitated movements, papules or vomiting of blood or nose bleeding, crimson tongue, yellow tongue moss, and rapid pulse.

These are symptoms of unresolved heat pathogens in the *qì* aspect and exuberant heat pathogens in the construction-blood aspect—of searing at both the *qì* and construction [blood] aspects. Vigorous fever, thirst, headache, and yellow tongue moss are characteristic of exuberant *qì* aspect heat. Crimson tongue, vexation, and agitation are characteristic of pathogenic heat harassing the heart construction. And papules, or vomiting of blood, or nose bleeding are caused by intensifying of blood heat.

The unique characteristic of this pattern is that it displays both *qì* aspect and construction-blood aspect symptoms. This makes it different from both intense *qì* aspect heat, and pathogenic heat entering the construction-blood aspect.

Treatment

Clear both the *qì* and construction (blood) aspects. Normally, Jade Lady Variant Brew (*Jiā Jiǎn Yù Nǚ Jiān*) can be used, but in serious cases Scourge-Clearing Toxin-Vanquishing Beverage (*Qīng Wēn Bài Dú Yǐn*) should be prescribed.

Prescriptions

Jade Lady Brew (*Yù Nǚ Jiān* 玉女煎)

—In which achyranthes [root] (*niú xī* 牛膝) and cooked rehmannia [root] (*shú dì* 熟地) have been replaced with thin raw rehmannia [root] (*xì shēng dì* 細生地) and Scrophularia [Root] Formula (*Xuán Shēn Fāng* 玄參方)—

From the *Detailed Analysis of Warm Diseases* (*Wēn Bìng Tiáo Biàn* 溫病條辯)

crude gypsum (*shēng shí gāo*)	生石膏	90g
anemarrhena [root] (*zhī mǔ*)	知母	12g
scrophularia [root] (*xuán shēn*)	玄參	12g
thin raw rehmannia [root] (*xì shēng dì*)	細生地	18g
ophiopogon [tuber] (*mài dōng*)	麥冬	18g

Boil the ingredients in eight cups of water until three cups are left. Divide into two doses. Keep the remnants and use them a second time.

This formula is a modification of Jǐng Yuè's Jade Lady Brew (*Yù Nǚ Jiān*). It contains:

- § Gypsum (*shí gāo*) and anemarrhena [root] (*zhī mǔ*), which clear *qì* aspect heat.
- § Scrophularia [root] (*xuán shēn*), raw rehmannia [root] (*shēng dì*), and ophiopogon [tuber] (*mài dōng*), which cool construction and enrich *yīn*.

Used together these medicinals clear *qì* and cool construction.

Scourge-Clearing Toxin-Vanquishing Beverage (*Qīng Wēn Bài Dú Yǐn* 清瘟敗毒飲)

From *Achievements Regarding Epidemic Papules* (*Yì Zhěn Yī Dé* 疫疹一得)

		LARGE	MEDIUM	SMALL
crude gypsum (*shēng shí gāo*) (boil first)	生石膏	180-240g	60-120g	24-36g
raw rehmannia [root] (*shēng dì huáng*)	生地黃	18-30g	10-15g	6-12g
rhinoceros horn (*xī jiǎo*)	犀角	18-24g	10-15g	6-12g
coptis [root] (*huáng lián*)	黃連	12-18g	6-12g	3-5g
gardenia [fruit] (*zhī zǐ*)	梔子	normal dose		
platycodon [root] (*jié gěng*)	桔梗	normal dose		
scutellaria [root] (*huáng qín*)	黃芩	normal dose		
anemarrhena [root] (*zhī mǔ*)	知母	normal dose		
red peony [root] (*chì sháo*)	赤芍	normal dose		
scrophularia [root] (*xuán shēn*)	玄參	normal dose		
forsythia [fruit] (*lián qiào*)	連翹	normal dose		
licorice [root] (*gān cǎo*)	甘草	normal dose		
moutan [root bark] (*dān pí*)	丹皮	normal dose		
bamboo leaf (*zhú yè*)	竹葉	normal dose		

These days, use 56-72g of water buffalo horn (*shuǐ niú jiǎo*) instead of 18-24g of rhinoceros horn (*xī jiǎo*). Grind the horn. Boil the gypsum (*shí gāo*), then add the other medicinals (including the ground horn) and administer when ready.

This formula is a modified combination of White Tiger Decoction (*Bái Hǔ Tāng*), Coptis Toxin-Resolving Decoction (*Huáng Lián Jiě Dú Tāng*), and Rhinoceros Horn and Rehmannia Decoction (*Xī Jiǎo Dì Huáng Tāng*). It therefore retains the functions of all three. It strongly clears *qì* and blood [aspect] heat, so it is called Scourge-Clearing Toxin-Vanquishing Beverage (*Qīng Wēn Bài Dú Yǐn*).

3. HEAT BINDING WITH BLOOD

Pattern

Hardness and fullness of the lower abdomen, black stools, manic episodes, sunken replete pulse, and blood stasis papules on the tongue.

These are symptoms of amassment of blood in the lower burner, and are usually seen when pathogens enter the blood aspect, heat and blood bind together, and amassments occur in the lower burner. Hardness and fullness of the lower abdomen results from heat and blood binding together in the lower burner, so in most cases pressure to the abdomen causes pain. The heart governs the blood, so when blood stasis blood aspect heat harasses the heart spirit there are manic episodes. The stools are black because there is blood stasis and the pulses are sunken and replete because pathogens are replete at the interior. Blood stasis obstructs internally, so there are blood stasis papules on the tongue.

Treatment

Attack below and discharge heat. Quicken blood and expel stasis.

Prescription

Peach Kernel Qì-Coordinating Decoction
(*Táo Rén Chéng Qì Tāng* 桃仁承氣湯)
From the *Detailed Analysis of Warm Diseases* (*Wēn Bìng Tiáo Biàn* 溫病條辯)

rhubarb (*dà huáng*)	大黄	15g
mirabilite (*máng xiāo*)	芒硝	6g
peach kernel (*táo rén*)	桃仁	10g
tangkuei (*dāng guī*)	當歸	10g
*peony [root] (*sháo yào*)	芍藥	10g
moutan [root bark] (*dān pí*)	丹皮	10g

*NOTE: In the case of this formula, peony [root] (*sháo yào*) can be taken to mean red peony [root] (*chì sháo*).

This formula is a modification of Peach Kernel Qì-Coordinating Decoction (*Táo Hé Chéng Qì Tāng*) from the *Treatise on Cold Damage*. Its overall aim is to downbear and eliminate both blood stasis and heat pathogens. It consists of:

§ Peach kernel (*táo rén*), moutan [root bark] (*dān pí*), red peony [root] (*chì sháo*), and tangkuei (*dāng guī*), which quicken and stir blood.

§ Rhubarb (*dà huáng*) and mirabilite (*máng xiāo*), which attack below, discharge heat, and throughclear stasis bind.

D. THE DISEASE PATTERN AND ITS TREATMENT IN EXUBERANT WIND-STIRRING HEAT

Pattern

Vigorous fever, dizzy head with pressure pain, (clonic) spasms of the four limbs and in severe cases tetanic reversal, manic derangement, red tongue with dry moss, and string-like rapid pulse.

These symptoms often occur during the course of diseases in which extreme heat engenders wind. Pathogenic heat is exuberant internally so there is vigorous fever. Extreme heat engenders wind, which harasses the clear orifices above, so there is dizzy head with pressure pain. The channel vessels are harassed so there are (clonic) spasms of the four limbs and in severe cases tetanic reversal. Heat harasses the spirit light so there is manic derangement. Exuberant heat damages the fluids so the tongue is red and the moss dry. Exuberant heat stirs liver wind internally so the pulse is string-like and rapid.

Treatment

Cool the liver and extinguish the wind.

Prescription

Antelope Horn and Uncaria Decoction
(*Líng Jiǎo Guō Téng Tāng* 羚角鈎藤湯)

From the *Popularized Treatise on Cold Damage* (*Tōng Sú Shāng Hán Lùn* 通俗傷寒論)

Antelope Horn Tablet (*Líng Jiǎo Piàn*) (cook first)	羚角片	5g
mulberry leaf (*sāng yè*)	桑葉	6g
Sichuan fritillaria [bulb] (*chuān bèi mǔ*) (remove the centers)	川貝母	12g
raw rehmannia [root] (*shēng dì*)	生地	15g
uncaria [stem and thorn] (*gōu téng*) (cook later)	鈎藤	10g

chrysanthemum [flower] (*jú huā*)	菊花	10g
root poria (*fú shén*)	茯神	10g
white peony [root] (*bái sháo*)	白芍	10g
raw licorice [root] (*shēng gān cǎo*)	生甘草	2g
fresh bamboo shavings (*xiān zhú rú*) (cook first)	鮮竹茹	15g

First, boil the Antelope Horn Tablet (*Líng Jiǎo Piàn*) and fresh bamboo shavings (*xiān zhú rú*) in about half a cup of water and set aside to drink separately. Then boil all the other medicinals in three cups of water until one cup is left. Keep the remnants and use them a second time.

In this formula:

§ Antelope horn (*líng yáng jiǎo*), uncaria [stem and thorn] (*gōu téng*), mulberry leaf (*sāng yè*), and chrysanthemum [flower] (*jú huā*) are used to cool the liver and extinguish wind.

§ Root poria (*fú shén*) is used to quiet the spirit and stabilize the mind.

§ Since heat condenses fluids into phlegm, fritillaria [bulb] (*bèi mǔ*) is used to transform phlegm.

§ Since effulgent fire engenders wind and wind fans fire, creating a vicious circle that renders the *yīn* fluids easily susceptible to damage, white peony [root] (*bái sháo*), licorice [root] (*gān cǎo*), and raw rehmannia [root] (*shēng dì*) are used for the *yīn* transforming and sinew- and vessel-enriching and nourishing actions of their sour and sweet flavors—to relax the sinew, vessel, and muscle spasms.

§ Bamboo shavings (*zhú rú*) are added to diffuse and through-clear the vessels and networks.

When these medicinals are combined, their overall effect is to cool the liver and extinguish the wind and increase the fluid and soothe the sinews. If there are accompanying symptoms of exuberant *qì* aspect heat, such as vigorous fever, copious sweating, and thirst with desire for cold drinks, add crude gypsum (*shēng shí gāo*) and anemarrhena [root] (*zhī mǔ*) to clear the *qì*. If there are accompanying symptoms of pathogens blocking the pericardium, such as clouded spirit and delirious speech, add Purple Snow Elixir (*Zǐ Xuě Dān*) to clear the heart, open the orifices, and extinguish the wind. If there are accompanying symptoms of bowel repletion, such as constipation, add rhubarb (*dà huáng*) and mirabilite (*máng xiāo*) to attack below and discharge heat. And, if there are accompanying symptoms of exuberant construction-blood aspect heat, such as crimson red tongue and rashes, add water buffalo horn (*shuǐ niú jiǎo*), raw rehmannia [root] (*shēng dì*), and moutan [root bark] (*dān pí*) to cool blood and resolve toxins.

E. DISEASE PATTERNS AND THEIR TREATMENTS IN HEAT SCORCHING THE TRUE YĪN

1. YĪN VACUITY WITH INTENSE HEAT

Pattern

Fever, vexation, restless sleep, red tongue, yellow moss, and fine rapid pulse.

These symptoms manifest when heat damages kidney *yīn* and exuberant heart fire flares. Heat pathogens enter lesser *yīn*, so heart fire flares above and kidney *yīn* vacates below. The more the *yīn* vacates, the more the fire flares; the more the fire flares, the more the *yīn* vacates. The more they respond to each other, the more they boost the disease. This causes vexation and restless sleep. As Wú Jú Tōng wrote, "(This is) flaring of *yáng*—*yáng* unable to enter *yīn*; *yīn* vacuity—*yīn* not receiving *yáng*." Fever, red tongue, yellow moss, and small rapid pulse result from exuberant *yīn* vacuity fire.

Treatment

Foster *yīn* and clear heat.

Prescription

Coptis and Ass Hide Glue Decoction
(*Huáng Lián Ē Jiāo Tāng* 黃連阿膠湯)

From the *Detailed Analysis of Warm Diseases* (*Wēn Bìng Tiáo Biàn* 溫病條辯)

coptis [root] (*huáng lián*)	黃連	12g
scutellaria [root] (*huáng qín*)	黃芩	3g
ass hide glue (*ē jiāo*)	阿膠	10g
white peony [root] (*bái sháo*)	白芍	3g
egg yolk (*jī zǐ huáng*)	鷄子黃	2 yokes

Boil all the ingredients except the ass hide glue (*ē jiāo*) and the egg yolk (*jī zǐ huáng*) in eight cups of water until three cups are left.

Remove the residue and stir the ass hide glue (*ē jiāo*) into the decoction until dissolved, and add the egg yolk (*jī zǐ huáng*). Give the decoction three times daily.

This prescription is the same as Coptis and Ass Hide Glue Decoction from the *Treatise on Cold Damage* except that the dosages have been altered. In it:

- Coptis [root] (*huáng lián*) and scutellaria [root] (*huáng qín*) clear pathogenic heat.
- Ass hide glue (*ē jiāo*), white peony [root] (*bái sháo*), and egg yolk (*jī zǐ huáng*) rescue true *yīn*.

When these medicinals are used together, their overall effect is to clear heat, foster *yīn*, and throughclear the heart and kidneys.

2. KIDNEY YĪN CONSUMED AND DETRIMENTED

Pattern

Lingering low fever, heat in the centers of the palms and soles, dry mouth, dry crimson-red tongue or in serious cases dry dark-purple tongue, lassitude of the spirit, deafness, and big vacuous pulse.

These symptoms are usually only seen during the final stages of a serious spring warmth disease. Warm diseases easily damage the *yīn* liquid, and chronically restrained pathogenic heat generally enters deeply into the lower burner where it robs and scorches the liver and kidney *yīn*. Consequently, pathogens are less prominent than vacuity.

Lingering low fever and heat in the centers of the palms and soles are characteristic of *yīn* vacuity with heat. Dry mouth and dry crimson-red tongue or in serious cases dry dark-purple tongue result from damaged liver and kidney *yīn*. The *yīn* essence is depleted and detrimented, and the right *qì* is vacuous and debilitated, so there is lassitude of the essence-spirit. The kidneys open into the ears, and the kidney essence is depleted and detrimented so there is deafness. Pathogens are less prominent than vacuity, so the pulse is big and without strength.

Treatment

Enrich the *yīn* and nourish the liquid.

Prescription

Pulse Restorative Variant Decoction
(*Jiā Jiǎn Fù Mài Tāng* 加減復脈湯)
From the *Detailed Analysis of Warm Diseases* (*Wēn Bìng Tiáo Biàn* 溫病條辯)

honey-fried licorice [root] (*zhì gān cǎo*)	炙甘草	18g
dried rehmannia [root] (*gān dì huáng*)	干地黃	18g
raw white peony [root] (*shēng bái sháo*)	生白芍	18g
ophiopogon [tuber] (*mài dōng*) (uncored)	麥冬	15g
ass hide glue (*ē jiāo*)	阿膠	10g
hemp seed (*má rén*)	麻仁	10g

Boil the ingredients in eight cups of water until three cups are left. Give three times daily. In serious cases use 30g of honey-fried licorice [root] (*zhì gān cǎo*), 24g each of raw rehmannia [root] (*shēng dì*) and raw white peony [root] (*shēng bái sháo*), and 21g of ophiopogon [tuber] (*mài dōng*). Give three times daily and once at night.

This prescription is a modification of Honey-Fried Licorice Decoction (*Zhì Gān Cǎo Tāng*) from the *Treatise on Cold Damage.* Ginseng (*rén shēn*), cinnamon twig (*guì zhī*), fresh ginger (*shēng jiāng*), and jujube (*dà zǎo*) have been replaced with raw white peony [root] (*shēng bái sháo*). It is the main prescription for warm disease pathogens entering the lower burner and damaging the liver and kidney *yīn*.

In this formula:

- Dried rehmannia [root] (*gān dì huáng*), ass hide glue (*ē jiāo*), raw white peony [root] (*shēng bái sháo*), and ophiopogon [tuber] (*mài dōng*) enrich the liver and kidney *yīn*.
- Honey-fried licorice [root] (*zhì gān cǎo*) supplements right *qì*.
- Hemp seed (*má rén*) moistens dryness.

When these medicinals are used together, their overall effect is to enrich *yīn* and abate heat, and nourish liquid and moisten dryness.

3. VACUITY WIND STIRRING INTERNALLY

Pattern

Severe fever and reversal, dry tongue and black teeth, cracked lips, sunken fine rapid pulse, twitching fingers, violent palpitations, or in serious cases lassitude of the spirit and chronic convulsions, vacuous pulse, crimson-red tongue, scant tongue moss, and constant verging on desertion.

This condition results from heat scorching the liver and kidney *yīn* and is characterized by symptoms of wind stirring internally. Heat consumes the true *yīn*, so pathogens are less prominent than vacuity. *Yīn* and *yáng qì* are not joining normally, so arm and leg reversal counterflow results. There is *yīn* vacuity internal heat, so the tongue is dry, the teeth are black, the lips are cracked, and the pulse is sunken, fine, and rapid. The true *yīn* is depleted and detrimented, so the liver loses nourishment, and there is stirring of vacuity wind internally with twitching fingers and violent palpitations. If the true *yīn* is further consumed and detrimented, vacuity wind tightens the body, causing lassitude of the spirit and chronic convulsions. Vacuous pulse, crimson red tongue, scant tongue moss, and constant verging on desertion are all symptoms of *yīn* and *yáng* separating.

This pattern [i.e., vacuity wind stirring internally] and the pattern of exuberant wind-stirring heat are both expressions of liver wind stirring internally, but in one the disease is vacuous, and in the other replete—so the symptoms of each are distinctly different. Exuberant wind-stirring heat can usually be seen during the heat abundant stage of a disease. It results from "extreme heat engendering wind," pertains to repletion, has the main symptom of strong (clonic) spasms in the four limbs, and is accompanied by vigorous fever, tetanic reversal, manic derangement, dry tongue moss, and thirst with desire to drink. Vacuity wind stirring internally, on the other hand, is usually seen during the final stages of a warm disease. It results from "blood vacuity engendering wind," pertains to vacuity, has the main symptom of twitching fingers or chronic convulsions, and is accompanied by black teeth, crimson-red tongue, scant tongue moss, vacuous pulse, and lassitude of the spirit. These two patterns are not difficult to distinguish. As Hé Xiù Shān (何秀山) comments:

> *Blood vacuity engendered wind is not true wind. Actually, it occurs because blood does not nourish sinews. Sinews and vessels are stiff, unable to extend and flex easily, so there are unremitting spasms of the hands and feet. Because it is like wind stirring it is called internal vacuity dim-wind. This pattern is generally only seen during the final stage of a warm heat disease, when blood and liquid are damaged by heat.*

Treatment

Nourish the *yīn* and extinguish the wind. Use Triple Armored Pulse-Restorative Decoction (*Sān Jiă Fù Mài Tāng*) or Major Wind-Stabilizing Pill (*Dà Dìng Fēng Zhū*).

Prescription

Triple Armored Pulse-Restorative Decoction
(*Sān Jiă Fù Mài Tāng* 三甲復脈湯)

From the *Detailed Analysis of Warm Diseases* (*Wēn Bìng Tiáo Biàn* 溫病條辯)

honey-fried licorice [root] (*zhì gān căo*)	炙甘草	18g
dried rehmannia [root] (*gān dì huáng*)	干地黃	18g
white peony [root] (*bái sháo*)	白芍	18g
ophiopogon [tuber] (*mài dōng*) (uncored)	麥冬	15g
ass hide glue (*ē jiāo*)	阿膠	10g
hemp seed (*má rén*)	麻仁	10g
crude oyster shell (*shēng mŭ lì*)	生牡蠣	15g
crude turtle shell (*shēng biē jiă*)	生鱉甲	18g
crude tortoise plastron (*shēng guī băn*)	生龜板	30g

Boil the ingredients in eight cups of water until three cups are left. Give as three doses over a single day.

Major Wind-Stabilizing Pill (*Dà Dìng Fēng Zhū* 大定風珠)

From the *Detailed Analysis of Warm Diseases* (*Wēn Bìng Tiáo Biàn* 溫病條辯)

raw white peony [root] (*shēng bái sháo*)	生白芍	18g
ass hide glue (*ē jiāo*)	阿膠	10g
crude tortoise plastron (*shēng guī băn*)	生龜板	12g
dried rehmannia [root] (*gān dì huáng*)	干地黃	18g
hemp seed (*má rén*)	麻仁	6g
schizandra [berry] (*wŭ wèi zĭ*)	五味子	6g
crude oyster shell (*shēng mŭ lì*)	生牡蠣	12g
ophiopogon [tuber] (*mài dōng*) (cored)	麥冬	18g
honey-fried licorice [root] (*zhì gān căo*)	炙甘草	12g
egg yolk (*jī zĭ huáng*)	鷄子黃	2 yolks
crude turtle shell (*shēng biē jiă*)	生鱉甲	12g

Boil all the ingredients except the egg yolk (*jī zĭ huáng*) in eight cups of water until three cups are left. Remove and discard the residue then stir in the egg yolk (*jī zĭ huáng*). Give thrice daily. For rapid respiration, add ginseng (*rén shēn*). For spontaneous sweating add dragon bone (*lóng gŭ*), ginseng (*rén shēn*), and wheat (*xiăo mài*). For palpitations add root poria (*fú shén*), ginseng (*rén shēn*), and wheat (*xiăo mài*).

Triple Armored Pulse-Restorative Decoction (*Sān Jiă Fù Mài Tāng*) is made by adding oyster shell (*mŭ lì*), crude turtle shell (*shēng biē jiă*), and crude tortoise plastron (*shēng guī băn*) to Pulse Restorative Variant Decoction (*Jiā Jiăn Fù Mài Tāng*). Pulse Restorative Variant Decoction is used to nourish the liver and kidney *yīn*. Oyster shell (*mŭ lì*), crude turtle shell (*shēng biē jiă*), and crude tortoise plastron (*shēng guī băn*) are added to extinguish wind and conceal *yáng*.

Major Wind-Stabilizing Pill (*Dà Dìng Fēng Zhū*) is made by adding egg yolk (*jī zĭ huáng*) and schizandra [berry] (*wŭ wèi zĭ*) to Triple Armored Pulse-Restorative Decoction. Egg yolk (*jī zĭ huáng*), a medicinal that resinates with flesh and blood, is added to nourish *yīn* and extinguish wind. Schizandra [berry] (*wŭ wèi zĭ*) is added to supplement *yīn*, constrain *yáng*, and curtail the possibility of reversal desertion.

F. THE DISEASE PATTERN AND ITS TREATMENT IN LINGERING PATHOGENS IN THE YĪN ASPECT

Pattern

Night fever that abates at dawn without sweating, good appetite but emaciated body.

These symptoms are generally seen when lingering residual pathogens are deep-seated in the construction *yīn* during the final stages of a spring warmth disease. Fever occurs at night, because construction *qì* resists pathogens and outpushes them to the *yáng* aspect. But it abates at dawn without sweating, because pathogens return to the *yīn* aspect without resolving the exterior. Since the pathogens are not in the *qì* aspect, the stomach and intestine functions are undiseased, and the appetite remains good. But because the construction *yīn* has been consumed and detrimented by the lingering residual pathogens and is therefore unable to nourish the muscles and skin, the body still becomes emaciated. As Wú Jú Tōng states:

> *Night time movement from the yīn aspect causing fever, and day time movement from the yáng aspect causing cold, means*

very deeply seated pathogenic qì in the yīn aspect. Fever abates without sweating because instead of moving out to the exterior, pathogens return to the yīn aspect.

Treatment

Nourish *yīn* and outthrust pathogens.

Prescriptions

Sweet Wormwood Turtle Shell Decoction
(*Qīng Hāo Bēi Jiă Tāng* 青蒿鱉甲湯)

From the *Detailed Analysis of Warm Diseases* (*Wēn Bìng Tiáo Biàn* 溫病條辯)

sweet wormwood (*qīng hāo*)	青蒿	6g
turtle shell (*biē jiă*)	鱉甲	15g
thin raw rehmannia [root] (*xì shēng dì*)	細生地	12g
anemarrhena [root] (*zhī mŭ*)	知母	6g
moutan [root bark] (*mŭ dān pí*)	牡丹皮	10g

Boil all the ingredients in five cups of water until two cups are left. Give twice daily.

In this prescription:

§ Sweet wormwood (*qīng hāo*), which is fragrant, outthrusts the network vessels and guides pathogens to the exterior.

§ Turtle shell (*biē jiă*) nourishes *yīn*, enters the network vessels and tracks pathogens.

§ Moutan [root bark] (*dān pí*) and raw rehmannia [root] (*shēng dì*) cool blood and nourish *yīn*.

§ Anemarrhena [root] (*zhī mŭ*) clears heat and regenerates liquid.

According to Wú Jú Tōng:

One of this formula's excellent features is that it can first enter and latter exit. Sweet wormwood (qīng hāo) is normally unable to enter the yīn aspect, but can be led in by turtle shell (biē jiă); turtle shell by itself, is unable to exit to the yáng aspect, but can be led out by sweet wormwood.

CHAPTER 9
SUMMERHEAT WARMTH

Summerheat warmth is an acute hot disease contracted during the summer season, and caused by summerheat-heat disease pathogens. It is marked by an abrupt onset and, during its initial stages, by characteristic qì aspect symptoms of vigorous fever, vexing thirst, and copious sweating. Moreover, its pathomechanism transmits and transmutes swiftly, readily damaging liquid and consuming *qì*, so after transmutation there are often symptoms of closed orifices and stirring wind. Summerheat warmth theory can be applied in pattern identification and treatment determination for biomedically defined conditions such as acute infectious encephalitis-B., leptospirosis, and heat stroke.

I. DISEASE CAUSES AND PATHOLOGY

Although the principal factor to which this disease can be attributed is an attack to the human body by a summerheat-heat disease pathogen, such an attack can only succeed provided there is also an insufficiency of right *qì*. It can only occur when hard physical labor during the extremely hot weather and abundant summerheat *qì* of summer consume and damage the liquid and *qì* causing a state of fatigue, or when there is a pre-existing depletion of right *qì* and summerheat pathogens then attack, while the human body is weakened. In the *Classic of Internal Medicine* it says, "*Qì* vacuity fever results from damage by summerheat." Lǐ Dōng Yuán (李東垣) explains this as follows:

Summerheat-heat is summer specific. When exhaustion resulting from hard work or undernourishment depletes original qì, people lack the strength to resist hot weather, so their bodies are damaged and diseases occur.

These passages show that the internal reason for this disease is an insufficiency of right *qì*, and the external reason is an attack by a summerheat-heat pathogen.

Summerheat is a type of fire heat *qì*, and as such it transmits and transmutes swiftly. When it attacks the human body it usually enters directly into the *qì* aspect, passing through the defense aspect without affecting it. Initially, symptoms of exuberant *yáng* brightness *qì* aspect heat such as high fever, vexing thirst, and copious sweating can be seen. So when Yè Tiān Shì stated, "Summer summerheat occurs at *yáng* brightness," he accurately summarized the characteristic onset of summerheat diseases. Summerheat has a harsh nature, so it can easily detriment and damage the right *qì*, and consume and detriment the fluids.

Therefore, during the course of this disease, it is quite possible that symptoms of serious damage such as damaged *qì* and consumed fluids or liquid *qì* verging on desertion will be seen. Also, summerheat has a scorching nature, so it can easily enter the heart construction and stir liver wind. In other words, unless timely action is taken to clear and resolve the *qì* aspect heat pathogen, it can easily transform into fire, and enter deeply into the heart construction where it can engender phlegm and engender wind. Under these circumstances, serious conditions like scorching of both the *qì* and construction [blood], phlegm-heat orifice closure, or wind and fire fanning each other can result. Such conditions are most commonly seen in children.

Although summerheat-heat is a *yáng* pathogen, when it causes disease it is often accompanied by a damp pathogen. Since summerheat *qì* is exuberant during summer, at which time there is also considerable damp *qì*, summerheat and dampness are usually contracted simultaneously—so symptoms of summerheat warmth harboring damp usually result. Apart from symptoms of summerheat-heat, there are also symptoms of stickiness caused by damp pathogen obstructions. Moreover, because the weather in summer is scorching hot and people like drinking cold drinks, summerheat warmth pathogens can easily be blocked by cold pathogens, and symptoms of summerheat-damp can occur with concurrent cold symptoms. Initially, the principal clinical manifestations are of simultaneous defense and *qì* aspects diseases.

During their final stages, summerheat diseases generally manifest as pathogenic heat slowly resolving and liquid *qì* not yet restoring. Clinically, there are symptoms of both liquid and *qì* vacuity, sometimes with simultaneous symptoms of intractable residual pathogenic *qì*. In the event that wind stirring blocks the orifices causing tetanic spasms and clouding of the spirit, after recovery, if phlegm-heat lodges in the envelope network vessels and blocks the orifices, there will be permanent residual symptoms of dulled wits, loss of speech, and deafness. Alternatively, if wind-phlegm attaches and stagnates in the channels and network vessels and prevents the tendon vessels from working properly, there will be tonic muscular contractions or extensions at the limbs, and in severe cases permanent paralysis.

II. MAIN POINTS OF DIAGNOSIS

1. Summerheat diseases usually occur during summer.

2. This type of disease has a rapid onset and is characterized initially by vigorous fever, copious sweating, vexing thirst, yellow tongue moss, and surging rapid pulse.

3. During the course of the disease, transformations are frequent and serious patterns of liquid *qì* verging on desertion, internal block, stirring of wind, or stirring of blood are quite commonly seen.

4. Accompanying symptoms of stomach duct dilations and slimy tongue moss are indicative of summerheat warmth with concurrent dampness and accompanying symptoms of aversion to cold and absence of sweating are indicative of summerheat-damp with concurrent cold.

III. PATTERN IDENTIFICATION AND TREATMENT DETERMINATION

Since summerheat is a fire heat pathogen, the principal treatment for this disease is to clear the summerheat and discharge the heat. But since summerheat easily damages *qì* and consumes liquid, as evidenced by the fact that wind stirring and closed orifices occur quite readily, it is commonly also treated with *qì*-boosting, fluid-engendering, orifice-opening, and wind-extinguishing methods. These methods are used according to the changes of the pathomechanism and symptom expressions during the disease process. The basic treatments are as follows:

1. During the initial stage of summerheat damage to the *qì* aspect with *yáng* brightness exuberant heat, use acrid cold medicinals to clear *qì*, discharge heat, and flush summerheat.

2. If summerheat-heat damages the fluids, use sweet cold medicinals to clear heat and engender liquid.

3. If summerheat-heat severely damages the body's liquid *qì* and then resolves, use sweet sour medicinals to boost the *qì* and constrain liquid.

As Zhāng Fèng Kuí (張鳳逵) wrote:

> *For summerheat disease first use acrid cool [medicinals], then use sweet cold [medicinals], then later use sweet sour [medicinals] to restrain the fluids. Downward directing medicinals must not be used.*

This passage summarizes the main treatment principles for the different stages of summerheat disease pathogens in the *qì* aspect. If summerheat-heat transforms into fire internally and passes to the heart construction, causing closed orifices and moving wind, use heart-clearing construction-cooling treatments, or phlegm-transforming orifice-opening treatments, or liver-cooling wind-extinguishing treatments according to the different conditions of the different patients. During the final stage of a summerheat disease in which the residual pathogens have not cleared and the *qì yīn* has not been restored, treat not only by boosting *qì* and nourishing *yīn*, but also by clearing and discharging residual heat.

If symptoms of summerheat and damp pathogens occur concurrently, use summerheat-clearing treatments and dampness-disinhibiting treatments concurrently. As Wáng Lún (王綸) said in his *Collection of Famous Míng Dynasty Doctors' Experiences* (*Míng Yī Zá Zhù* 明醫雜著), "Of all the summerheat treatment methods, the best is clearing the heart and disinhibiting the urine." This passage advocates the summerheat-clearing dampness-disinhibiting method. If summerheat-damp is obstructed by cold, clear the summerheat and transform the dampness, while concurrently resolving the exterior and scattering the cold.

A. DISEASE PATTERNS AND THEIR TREATMENTS IN DISEASES THAT ORIGINATE AS SUMMERHEAT

1. SUMMERHEAT ENTERING YÁNG BRIGHTNESS

Pattern

High fever and vexation, headache and dizziness, red complexion and rough breathing, thirst and copious sweating or slight aversion to cold in the back, dry yellow tongue moss, and surging rapid or surging big scallion-stalk pulse.

These symptoms are characteristic of summerheat-heat injuring *qì*, searing and intensifying in *yáng* brightness. *Yáng* brightness channel heat bellows steam so there is high fever, and its fumes harass internally so there is vexation. Heat steams upward to the head and eyes so there is headache, dizziness, and red complexion. Liquid is forced to discharge externally so there is copious sweating and thirst. The *qì* dynamic is congested internally so there is rough breathing. Dry yellow tongue moss and surging rapid pulse are characteristics of exuberant *yáng* brightness heat. In short, these are all exuberant heat, *yáng* brightness, *qì* aspect, replete external and internal symptoms. When slight aversion to cold in the back and surging big scallion-stalk pulse occur, they indicate that steaming of summerheat-heat has discharged too much sweating, and that right *qì* has been damaged. This type of aversion to cold is very different from the aversion to cold without sweating seen in external patterns.

Treatment

Clear summerheat and discharge heat. If the liquid qì has been damaged, simultaneously boost qì and engender liquid.

Prescriptions

White Tiger Decoction (*Bái Hŭ Tāng* 白虎湯)
From the *Treatise on Cold Damage* (*Shāng Hán Lùn* 傷寒論)

anemarrhena [root] (*zhī mŭ*)	知母	180g
gypsum (*shí gāo*)	石膏	500g
honey-fried licorice [root] (*zhì gān căo*)	炙甘草	60g
round-grained nonglutinous rice (*jīng mĭ*)	粳米	6 handfuls

Boil all four ingredients in one deciliter of water and cook until the round-grained nonglutinous rice (*jīng mĭ*) is ready, remove the residue and give the decoction in one-liter doses, while still warm, three times per day.

White Tiger Decoction Plus Ginseng
(*Bái Hŭ Jiā Rén Shēn Tāng* 白虎加人參湯)
From the *Detailed Analysis of Warm Diseases* (*Wēn Bìng Tiáo Biàn* 溫病條辯)

gypsum (*shí gāo*)	石膏	30g
anemarrhena [root] (*zhī mŭ*)	知母	15g
licorice [root] (*gān căo*)	甘草	10g
round-grained nonglutinous rice (*jīng mĭ*)	粳米	12g
ginseng (*rén shēn*)	人參	10g

Boil all the ingredients in eight cups of water until three cups are left. Give thrice daily. If the condition improves, reduce the dosage but continue the medication. If not, continue to administer the same dosage.

When summerheat enters *yáng* brightness, since the heat is both external and internal, White Tiger Decoction (*Bái Hŭ Tāng*) is prescribed. It is used to clear summerheat, discharge heat, and outthrust pathogens. If a *yáng* brightness pathogen fails to resolve and damages liquid *qì*, not only must treatment aim primarily to clear heat, but secondarily to boost *qì*. White Tiger Decoction Plus Ginseng (*Bái Hŭ Jiā Rén Shēn Tāng*) is appropriate because White Tiger Decoction (*Bái Hŭ Tāng*) clears summerheat and discharges heat, and ginseng (*rén shēn*) boosts *qì* and engenders liquid.

2. LIQUID *QÌ* DAMAGED BY SUMMERHEAT

Pattern

Fever, high breathing, vexation, yellow urine, thirst, spontaneous sweating, fatigued limbs, wearied spirit, and weak vacuous pulse.

This pattern is characteristic of summerheat-heat detrimenting and damaging liquid-*qì*. Summerheat-heat is confined internally so there is fever, high breathing, vexation, and yellow urine. The fluids are damaged so there is thirst. The original *qì* is depleted and detrimented so there are fatigued limbs with wearied spirit and spontaneous sweating. When all of these symptoms are considered together they indicate relatively exuberant summerheat-heat and damaged liquid *qì*. In comparison to summerheat entering *yáng* brightness, the heat pathogen is less severe but the fluids are more detrimented and damaged.

Treatment

Clear heat and flush summerheat. Boost *qì* and engender liquid.

Prescription

Wáng's Summerheat-Clearing Qì-Boosting Decoction
(*Wáng Shì Qīng Shǔ Yì Qì Tāng* 王氏清暑益氣湯)
From *Warm Heat Latitudes and Longitudes* (*Wēn Rè Jīng Wěi* 温热经纬)

American ginseng (*xī yáng shēn*)	西洋參	10g
dendrobium [stem] (*shí hú*)	石斛	10g
ophiopogon [tuber] (*mài dōng*)	麥冬	6g
coptis [root] (*huáng lián*)	黃連	2.5g
bamboo leaf (*zhú yè*)	竹葉	10g
lotus stalk (*hé gěng*)	荷梗	10g
anemarrhena [root] (*zhī mǔ*)	知母	10g
licorice [root] (*gān cǎo*)	甘草	3g
round-grained nonglutinous rice (*jīng mǐ*)	粳米	10g
watermelon rind (*xī guā cuì yī*)	西瓜翠衣	12g

Boil all the ingredients in water and drink while still warm.

When this pattern occurs, since the summerheat pathogen has not cleared, aim principally to clear summerheat, but since liquid *qì* has also been damaged, aim secondary to boost *qì* and engender liquid.

In Wáng's Summerheat-clearing Qì-Boosting Decoction (*Wáng Shì Qīng Shǔ Yì Qì Tāng*):

§ American ginseng (*xī yáng shēn*), dendrobium [stem] (*shí hú*), licorice [root] (*gān cǎo*), and polished round-grained nonglutinous rice (*jīng mǐ*) boost *qì* and engender liquid.

§ Coptis [root] (*huáng lián*), anemarrhena [root] (*zhī mǔ*), bamboo leaf (*zhú yè*), lotus stalk (*hé gěng*), and watermelon rind (*xī guā cuì yī*) clear heat and flush summerheat.

Compared with White Tiger Decoction (*Bái Hǔ Tāng*) and White Tiger Decoction Plus Ginseng (*Bái Hǔ Jiā Rén Shēn Tāng*), it is not as good at clearing heat and boosting *qì*, but better at engendering liquid.

3. LIQUID *QÌ* VERGING ON DESERTION

Pattern

Diminishing fever, non-stop sweating, panting, verging on desertion, and scattered big pulse.

This pattern occurs when the liquid *qì* has been damaged and consumed, the *qì* is vacuous and there is verging on desertion. The pathogenic *qì* has abated but the right *qì*, having been consumed and scattered, is unable to govern containment, so fluid discharges externally and there is non-stop sweating even though fever is diminishing. The liquid has been damaged and the *qì* has been consumed, so the transformation source of the lung is verging on exhaustion—there is panting, verging on desertion, and scattered big pulse. In this pattern sweating, consumption of liquid *qì*, damage to right *qì*, and discharge of sweating are all relatively severe. Therefore, although different from both of the *yáng* vacuity desertion patterns, it still presents a critical condition.

Treatment

Boost *qì* and constrain liquid. Engender the pulse and curtail desertion.

Prescription

Pulse-Engendering Powder (*Shēng Mài Sǎn* 生脈散)
From the *Detailed Analysis of Warm Diseases* (*Wēn Bìng Tiáo Biàn* 溫病條辯)

ginseng (*rén shēn*)	人參	10g
ophiopogon [tuber] (*mài mén dōng*)	麥門冬	6g
schizandra [berry] (*wǔ wèi zǐ*)	五味子	3g

Boil the ingredients in three cups of water until two cups are left. Divide the decoction into two doses, retain the residue and later boil it again. If the pulse does not return, keep administering the same prescription until it does.

Since the key pathomechanisms in this pattern are liquid damage and *qì* desertion, *qì*-boosting and desertion-curtailing treatment must be administered without delay. Pulse-Engendering Powder (*Shēng Mài Săn*) combines ginseng (*rén shēn*), which is used to benefit original *qì*, with sour sweet ophiopogon [tuber] (*mài mén dōng*), and schizandra [berry] (*wŭ wèi zĭ*), which are used to engender *yīn*. When the original *qì* is restrained, sweating is unable to discharge externally—*yīn* humor confines itself internally so *qì* is restrained. According to Xú Líng Tāi (徐靈胎):

> *Pulse-Engendering Powder is a formula used for deep seated summerheat damage to the fluids. Before it can be used care must be taken to determine whether or not there is pathogenic qì. Do not make the mistake of thinking that it is suitable for the treatment of summerheat.*

This formula cannot be used in cases where liquid *qì* has been damaged but summerheat-heat has not been cleared, or the consequential retention of pathogens causes future complications.

4. SUMMERHEAT INJURING THE HEART AND KIDNEYS

Pattern

Heart heat with vexation and agitation, non-stop wasting-thirst, crimson-red tongue, and dry yellow tongue moss.

This pattern is characteristic of summerheat-heat lingering in the *qì* aspect with residual pathogens affecting the heart and kidneys. Such inabilities of water and fire to communicate are usually seen during the late stage of summerheat warm diseases. There is residual heat harassing the heart so there is heart heat with vexation and agitation. There is intense flaring of heart fire so the spirit mind is not quiet. The kidney *yīn* has been scorched by heat and the *yīn* humor is unable to press upward so there is non-stop wasting-thirst. Crimson-red tongue and dry yellow tongue moss are both manifestations of damaged *yīn* and heat confinement.

Treatment

Clear heart fire and nourish kidney water.

Prescription

Coptis and Mume Decoction (*Lián Méi Tāng* 連梅湯) From the *Detailed Analysis of Warm Diseases* (*Wēn Bìng Tiáo Biàn* 溫病條辯)		
coptis [root] (*huáng lián*)	黃連	6g
mume [fruit] (*wū méi*) (remove the stones)	烏梅	10g
ophiopogon [tuber] (*mài dōng*) (remove the cores)	麥冬	10g
raw rehmannia [root] (*shēng dì*)	生地	10g
ass hide glue (*ē jiāo*)	阿膠	6g

Boil all the ingredients in four cups of water until two cups are left. Give in two separate doses. If the pulse is vacuous, big, and scallion-stalk, add ginseng (*rén shēn*).

The key pathomechanism of these symptoms is intense exuberance of heart fire with kidney water not communicating. This establishes a vicious circle—the more the heart fire intensifies, the more the kidney water is damaged; the more the kidney water depletes, the more the heart fire intensifies. Coptis and Mume Decoction (*Lián Méi Tāng*) is prescribed to clear the heart and drain the fire, and enrich the kidney and nourish the *yīn*.

This formula is a modification of Coptis and Ass Hide Glue Decoction (*Huáng Lián Ē Jiāo Tāng*). In it:

- Coptis [root] (*huáng lián*) clears the heart and drains fire.
- Ass hide glue (*ē jiāo*) and raw rehmannia [root] (*shēng dì*) enrich the kidney and nourish *yīn*.
- Ophiopogon [tuber] (*mài dōng*), which is sweet and cold, engenders liquid.
- Mume [fruit] (*wū méi*), which is bitter and sour, discharges heat.

When the sweet and sour flavors are combined they are able to transform *yīn*. When heart fire clears, kidney humor restores and the symptoms of heart heat, vexation, and wasting-thirst disappear.

5. SUMMERHEAT DAMAGING THE LUNG NETWORK VESSELS

Pattern

Sudden expectoration of blood, nose bleeding, coughing and rough breathing, lack of mental and visual clarity, scorching heat with vexation and thirst, red tongue, yellow tongue moss, and wiry rapid pulse.

This pattern results from summerheat-heat pathogen toxins invading the lung viscera and damaging its *yáng* network vessels, so its principal clinical manifestations are sudden expectoration of blood and coughing. Moreover, since these and the main symptoms of consumption (i.e., lung tuberculosis) are the same, this pattern is sometimes referred to as "summerheat consumption."

Summerheat-heat damages the lungs and detriments the *yáng* network vessels so blood floods out above causing sudden expectoration of blood and nose bleeding. Heat congests the lung *qi* leading to loss of depurative downbearing so there is coughing and rough breathing. Distressful steaming of summerheat-heat causes scorching heat with vexation and thirst, plus lack of mental and visual clarity. Red tongue, yellow tongue moss, and string-like rapid pulse are characteristic of internally exuberant summerheat-heat. These symptoms have a very sudden onset and are very serious. In severe cases, expectoration of blood is profuse and blood runs from the nose like water from a tap. Sometimes, when loss of blood is too severe, there can even be *qì* deserting with the blood.

Treatment

Clear heat and resolve toxins. Cool blood and stop bleeding. Use Rhinoceros Horn and Rehmannia Decoction (*Xī Jiǎo Dì Huáng Tāng* 犀角地黃湯) plus Lonicera and Forsythia Powder (*Yín Qiào Sǎn* 銀翹散).

Prescriptions

Rhinoceros Horn and Rehmannia Decoction
(*Xī Jiǎo Dì Huáng Tāng* 犀角地黃湯)
From the *Detailed Analysis of Warm Diseases* (*Wēn Bìng Tiáo Biàn* 溫病條辯)

dried rehmannia [root] (*gān dì huáng*)	干地黃	30g
raw white peony [root] (*shēng bái sháo*)	生白芍	10g
moutan [root bark] (*dān pí*)	丹皮	10g
rhinoceros horn (*xī jiǎo*)	犀角	10g

These days, use 30g of water buffalo horn (*shuǐ niú jiǎo*) instead of 10g of rhinoceros horn (*xī jiǎo*). Boil in five cups of water until two cups are left. Give twice daily. Keep the remnants and use again.

Lonicera and Forsythia Powder (*Yín Qiào Săn* 銀翹散) From the *Detailed Analysis of Warm Diseases* (*Wēn Bìng Tiáo Biàn* 溫病條辯)		
lonicera [flower] (*jīn yín huā*)	金銀花	10g
forsythia [fruit] (*lián qiào*)	連翹	10g
platycodon [root] (*jié gĕng*)	桔梗	6g
arctium [seed] (*niú bàng zĭ*) (crush)	牛蒡子	10g
mint (*bò hé*) (add later)	薄荷	6g
fermented soybean (*dòu chĭ*)	豆豉	10g
schizonepeta (*jīng jiè*)	荆芥	12g
bamboo leaf (*dàn zhú yè*)	淡竹葉	10g
raw licorice [root] (*shēng gān căo*)	生甘草	6g

Combine all the ingredients, grind them into powder, divide the powder into six-gram doses, and boil each dose with fresh phragmites [root] (*xiān lú gēn*). Decoctions should be administered quickly, as soon as they start giving off an aroma.

When summerheat-heat damages the lung, the main aims of therapy must be to safeguard the lung by clearing the summerheat-heat and to stop bleeding by clearing network vessel heat. Use Rhinoceros Horn and Rehmannia Decoction (*Xī Jiăo Dì Huáng Tāng*) as the principal prescription to cool blood, resolve toxins, clear the network vessels, and stop bleeding, and add modified Lonicera and Forsythia Powder (*Yín Qiào Săn*) to diffuse the lung and clear the heat. Since there is no need to outthrust the exterior, omit fermented soybean (*dòu chĭ*), schizonepeta (*jīng jiè*), and mint (*bò hé*), and consider replacing them with supplements like gardenia [fruit] (*shān zhī*), scutellaria [root] (*huáng qín*), imperata [root] (*máo gēn*), and biota leaf (*cè băi yè*), which clear heat and drain fire, cool blood and stop bleeding.

6. WIND-STIRRING SUMMERHEAT-HEAT

Pattern

Scorching heat, convulsion of the limbs and sometimes arched-back rigidity, clenched jaw, confounded unclear spirit, possibly phlegm congestion in the throat, and rapid string-like pulse.

This pattern results from intensely exuberant summerheat-heat stirring liver wind. Consequently, it is sometimes called "summerheat wind." Summerheat is a fire heat pathogen, which when it enters the human body can easily fall into reverting *yīn*, stir liver wind, and cause tetanic reversal. The principal manifestations of this pattern—scorching heat, convulsion of the limbs, and sometimes arched-back rigidity, clenched jaw, and rapid string-like pulse—are all expressions of exuberant wind-stirring heat. Confounded unclear spirit occurs when mutual exacerbation of wind and fire harass and derange the spirit light. If there is phlegm congestion in the throat, then wind stirring has engendered phlegm, which has followed fire upward and congested.

These symptoms are seen in summerheat warm diseases, and also in summerheat-heat stroke—the highest incidence of which occurs amongst children. According to Wú Jú Tōng, "When children affected by summerheat warmth have symptoms of fever and sudden tetanic reversion, their condition is called 'summerheat epilepsy'." Summerheat wind and summerheat epilepsy are actually two different names for the same disease.

Treatment

Clear heat and extinguish wind.

Prescription

Antelope Horn and Uncaria Decoction
(*Líng Jiǎo Gōu Téng Tāng* 羚角鈎藤湯)
From *Popularized Treatise on Cold Damage* (*Tōng Sú Shāng Hán Lùn* 通俗傷寒論).

antelope horn (*líng yáng jiǎo*) (cook first)	羚羊角	5g
mulberry leaf (*sāng yè*)	桑葉	6g
fritillaria [bulb] (*bèi mǔ*) (remove the centers)	貝母	12g
raw rehmannia [root] (*shēng dì*)	生地	15g
uncaria [stem and thorn] (*gōu téng*) (cook later)	鈎藤	10g
chrysanthemum [flower] (*jú huā*)	菊花	10g
root poria (*fú shén*)	茯神	10g
white peony [root] (*bái sháo*)	白芍	10g
raw licorice [root] (*shēng gān cǎo*)	生甘草	2g
fresh bamboo shavings (*xiān zhú rú*) (cook first)	鮮竹茹	15g

First, boil the antelope horn (*líng yáng jiǎo*) and fresh bamboo shavings (*xiān zhú rú*) together in about half a cup of water and set the decoction aside to drink separately. Then boil all the other ingredients in three cups of water until one cup is left. Keep the remnants and use them a second time.

This pattern occurs when exuberant heat stirs liver wind, so use Antelope Horn and Uncaria Decoction (*Líng Jiăo Gōu Téng Tāng*) to clear heat, cool the liver, extinguish wind, and settle spasms. For intense exuberance of *yáng* brightness *qì* aspect heat add gypsum (*shí gāo*) and anemarrhena [root] (*zhī mŭ*), which are acrid and cold, to clear the *qì*. For dryness bind bowel repletion, add rhubarb (*dà huáng*) and mirabilite (*máng xiāo*) to throughclear the bowels and discharge heat. For exuberant heart construction heat add water buffalo horn (*shuĭ niú jiăo*) and scrophularia [root] (*xuán shēn*) to clear construction and discharge heat. For pathogens blocking the pericardium add Purple Snow Elixir (*Zĭ Xuĕ Dān*) to extinguish wind and open the orifices. For strong heat and exuberant toxins add isatis root (*băn lán gēn*) and isatis leaf (*dà qīng yè*) to clear heat and resolve toxins. For phlegm-drool congestion add bile-processed arisaema [root] (*dăn nán xīng*) and bamboo sugar (*zhú huáng*) to clear and transform phlegm-heat. And for intractable repetitious convulsions add scorpion (*quán xiē*) and earthworm (*dì lóng*) to help stabilize the tetany.

7. SUMMERHEAT ENTERING HEART CONSTRUCTION

Pattern

Scorching heat with vexation and agitation, restless sleep, sometimes delirious speech or even coma, crimson-red tongue, and fine rapid pulse. Alternatively there can be sudden clouding collapse with loss of consciousness, fever, cold limbs, rough breathing, slightly tight jaw or closed mouth, crimson tongue, and rapid pulse.

Summerheat is a fire heat pathogen and as such it transmits and transmutes very quickly. When it enters the human body, it usually enters directly into the *qì* aspect, and easily falls into the heart construction. As our predecessors have therefore said, "summerheat easily enters the heart." Summerheat entering the heart construction can be seen during summerheat warm diseases, but can also occur in sudden clouding reversal—where summerheat-heat blocks the pericardium internally. In clinical practice, this is called summerheat reversal.

Summerheat-heat enters the construction where it harasses and deranges the heart spirit, so there is scorching heat with vexation and agitation, and sometimes delirious speech. The heat pathogen falls into the pericardium, where it clouds and blocks the clear orifice, so there is delirious speech or sometimes even coma. Crimson-red tongue and fine rapid pulse are both characteristic symptoms of heat harassing the heart construction and fire scorching the *yīn* construction.

If summerheat-heat pathogens attack the human body abruptly and block the pericardium internally, there is sudden clouding collapse with loss of consciousness. And since summerheat-heat simultaneously distresses internally, there is accompanying fever and rough breathing. In addition, the *yáng* is confined—unable to outpush to the four limbs so the four limbs suffer reversal cold. This pattern and wind stroke are similar in that they both occur very suddenly. Wind stroke however is usually characterized by accompanying Bell's palsy, whereas this pattern is not. Also, this disease is usually only seen during the hottest parts of summer when summerheat is particularly harsh. Wind stroke and summerheat stroke are therefore not difficult to differentiate.

Treatment

Cool construction and discharge heat. Clear the heart and open the orifices.

Prescriptions

Construction-Clearing Decoction (*Qīng Yíng Tāng* 清營湯)

From the *Detailed Analysis of Warm Diseases* (*Wēn Bìng Tiáo Biàn* 溫病條辯)

rhinoceros horn (*xī jiǎo*)	犀角	10g
raw rehmannia [root] (*shēng dì*)	生地	15g
scrophularia [root] (*xuán shēn*)	玄參	15g
tender bamboo leaf (*zhú yè xīn*)	竹葉心	3g
ophiopogon [tuber] (*mài dōng*)	麥冬	10g
salvia [root] (*dān shēn*)	丹參	6g
coptis [root] (*huáng lián*)	黃連	5g
lonicera [flower] (*jīn yín huā*)	金銀花	10g
forsythia [fruit] (*lián qiào*) (uncored)	連翹	6g

These days, use 30g of water buffalo horn (*shuǐ niú jiǎo*) instead of 10g of rhinoceros horn (*xī jiǎo*). Boil all the ingredients in eight cups of water until three cups are left. Give in one cup doses three times daily.

Peaceful Palace Bovine Bezoar Pill
(*Ān Gōng Niú Huáng Wán* 安宮牛黃丸)
From the *Detailed Analysis of Warm Diseases* (*Wēn Bìng Tiáo Biàn* 溫病條辯)

bovine bezoar (*niú huáng*)	牛黃	30g
curcuma [tuber] (*yù jīn*)	鬱金	30g
rhinoceros horn (*xī jiǎo*)	犀角	30g
coptis [root] (*huáng lián*)	黃連	30g
cinnabar (*zhū shā*)	朱砂	30g
borneol (*bīng piàn*)	冰片	8g
musk (*shè xiāng*)	麝香	8g
pearl (*zhēn zhū*)	珍珠	15g
gardenia [fruit] (*shān zhī*)	山梔	30g
realgar (*xióng huáng*)	雄黃	30g
scutellaria [root] (*huáng qín*)	黃芩	30g

These days, use 90g of water buffalo horn (*shuǐ niú jiǎo*) instead of 30g of rhinoceros horn (*xī jiǎo*). Grind into powder, combine with honey, and press into three-gram pills. Then cover with goldleaf and protect with wax. Give three doses per day.

Initially, when heat has entered the construction but has not yet blocked the orifices by stirring the blood, use Construction-Clearing Decoction (*Qīng Yíng Tāng*), which clears construction and discharges heat, as the principal remedy. This formula outthrusts the pathogen from the construction aspect to the *qì* aspect and resolves it. Later, when the heat pathogen has fallen into the pericardium, use Peaceful Palace Bovine Bezoar Pill (*Ān Gōng Niú Huáng Wán*) to clear the heart and open the orifices. Whenever attacks of summerheat-heat pathogens block and close the clear orifices causing sudden clouding reversal, take emergency measures to clear the heart and open the orifices.

Prescriptions like Peaceful Palace Bovine Bezoar Pill (*Ān Gōng Niú Huáng Wán*) must be administered or acupuncture must be used at points such as Human Middle (*rén zhōng*, GV-26), the ten diffusing points (*shí xuān*), Marsh at the Bend (*qū zé*, LI-11), and Uniting Bones (*hé gǔ*, LI-4) to arouse the spirit mind and to clear and discharge pathogenic heat. If the spirit has been cleared and the reversal has returned, but there are residual summerheat-heat pathogens in the *qì* and construction aspects, use *qì*-clearing summerheat-flushing or construction-clearing *yīn*-nourishing prescriptions.

8. SUMMERHEAT ENTERING THE BLOOD ASPECT

Pattern

Scorching heat with agitation and harassment, purple-black rashes, vomiting blood, nose bleeding, clouded spirit and delirious raving, in severe cases convulsions of the four limbs or arched-back rigidity, phlegm gurgling in the throat, crimson-red tongue, and charred tongue moss.

In this pattern, extremely exuberant summerheat-heat fire toxins sear and scorch the blood aspect and fall into the pericardium. Wind stirs, phlegm engenders, and the disease dynamic is very dangerous. The symptoms of scorching heat, agitation and harassment, and stupor and delirious speech are characteristic of construction-blood heat toxins searing intensely, blocking the pericardium internally, and confusing the heart spirit, whereas the symptoms of rashes and vomiting of blood are characteristic of exuberant blood aspect heat compelling frenetic movement of blood. Since heat is exuberant, it tends to stir liver wind, and wind stirring tends to engender phlegm. When this occurs, accompanying symptoms of convulsions are usually seen. Phlegm gurgling in the throat is characteristic of liver wind stirring internally and turbid phlegm congesting above.

Treatment

Cool blood and resolve toxins. Clear the heart and open the orifices.

Prescriptions

Spirit-Like Rhinoceros Horn Elixir (*Shén Xī Dān* 神犀丹)

From *Warm Heat Latitudes and Longitudes* (*Wēn Rè Jīng Wěi* 温热经纬)

rhinoceros horn tip (*xī jiăo jiān*) (grind in water)	犀角尖	180g
acorus [root] (*shí chāng pú*)	石菖蒲	180g
scutellaria [root] (*huáng qín*)	黄芩	180g
purified feces (*fèn qīng*)	糞清	300g
forsythia [fruit] (*lián qiào*)	連翹	300g
raw rehmannia [root] (*shēng dì*) (use fresh juice)	生地	450g
lonicera [flower] (*jīn yín huā*) (use fresh juice)	金銀花	450g
isatis root (*băn lán gēn*)	板籃根	270g
fermented soybean (*dòu chǐ*)	豆豉	240g
scrophularia [root] (*xuán shēn*)	玄參	210g
trichosanthes root (*huā fěn*)	花粉	120g
puccoon (*zǐ căo*)	紫草	120g

These days, use 540g of water buffalo horn (*shuĭ niú jiăo*) instead of 180g of rhinoceros horn (*xī jiăo*), and omit purified feces (*fèn qīng*). First grind the water buffalo horn (*shuĭ niú jiăo*) in water, and extract the juices from the raw rehmannia [root] (*shēng dì*) and lonicera [flower] (*jīn yín huā*). Then grind all the remaining ingredients into a powder and form it into pills using the liquid from grinding the water buffalo horn (*shuĭ niú jiăo*) and the juices from the raw rehmannia [root] (*shēng dì*) and lonicera [flower] (*jīn yín huā*). Do not use honey. If it is hard to form pills, add fermented soybean (*dòu chĭ*). Each pill should weigh nine grams.

Peaceful Palace Bovine Bezoar Pill
(*Ān Gōng Niú Huáng Wán* 安宫牛黄丸)
From the *Detailed Analysis of Warm Diseases* (*Wēn Bìng Tiáo Biàn* 溫病條辯)

bovine bezoar (*niú huáng*)	牛黄	30g
curcuma [tuber] (*yù jīn*)	鬱金	30g
rhinoceros horn (*xī jiăo*)	犀角	30g
coptis [root] (*huáng lián*)	黄連	30g
cinnabar (*zhū shā*)	朱砂	30g
borneol (*bīng piàn*)	冰片	8g
musk (*shè xiāng*)	麝香	8g
pearl (*zhēn zhū*)	珍珠	15g
gardenia [fruit] (*shān zhī*)	山梔	30g
realgar (*xióng huáng*)	雄黄	30g
scutellaria [root] (*huáng qín*)	黄芩	30g

These days, use 90g of water buffalo horn (*shuĭ niú jiăo*) instead of 30g of rhinoceros horn (*xī jiăo*). Grind all the ingredients into powder, combine with honey, and press into three-gram pills. Cover with goldleaf and protect with wax. Give three doses per day.

When exuberant wind-stirring heat causes convulsions of the four limbs, add antelope horn (*líng yáng jiăo*) and uncaria [stem and thorn] (*gōu téng*) or Tetany-Relieving Powder (*Zhĭ Jìng Săn* 止痙散), which contains scorpion (*quán xiē*), centipede (*wú gōng*), and silkworm (*jiāng cán*).

For phlegm congestion, add bamboo sugar (*tiān zhú huáng*), bile-processed arisaema [root] (*dăn nán xīng*), and dried bamboo sap (*zhú lì*), or Macaque Stone Powder (*Hóu Zăo Săn* 猴棗散), containing antelope horn (*líng yáng jiăo*), musk (*shè xiāng*), macaque stone (*hóu zăo*), calcine borax (*duàn yuè shí*), resinous aquilaria [wood] (*qié nán xiāng*), Sichuan fritillaria [bulb] (*chuān bèi mŭ*), chlorite (*qīng méng shí*) and bamboo sugar (*tiān zhú huáng*).

The symptoms of summerheat entering the blood aspect are more severe than those of the previous pattern (i.e., summerheat entering the heart construction), so during treatment it is essential that large doses of heat-clearing toxin-resolving medicinals and blood-cooling orifice-opening medicinals be used.

Spirit-Like Rhinoceros Horn Elixir (*Shén Xī Dān*) contains:

§ Water buffalo horn (*shuǐ niú jiǎo*), scutellaria [root] (*huáng qín*), lonicera [flower] (*jīn yín huā*), forsythia [fruit] (*lián qiào*), scrophularia [root] (*xuán shēn*), and isatis root (*bǎn lán gēn*), to cool blood and resolve toxins.

§ Raw rehmannia [root] (*shēng dì*), puccoon (*zǐ cǎo*), and fermented soybean (*dòu chǐ*), to cool blood and outthrust papules.

§ Trichosanthes root (*tiān huā fěn*), to engender liquid and stop thirst.

§ Acorus [root] (*shí chāng pú*), to open the orifices with aroma.

Peaceful Palace Bovine Bezoar Pill (*Ān Gōng Niú Huáng Wán*) is added to strengthen the orifice-opening action and rouse the spirit. When wind stirring causes convulsions, antelope horn (*líng yáng jiǎo*) and uncaria [stem and thorn] (*gōu téng*) are added to cool the liver and extinguish wind, or Tetany-Relieving Powder (*Zhǐ Jìng Sǎn*) is added to strengthen the tetany-stopping function. When exuberant phlegm-drool becomes congested, medicinals such as bamboo sugar (*tiān zhú huáng*), bile-processed arisaema [root] (*dǎn nán xīng*), dried bamboo sap (*zhú lì*), and/or Macaque Stone Powder (*Hóu Zǎo Sǎn*) are added to remove congested phlegm from the airways by clearing and transforming phlegm-heat. This prevents *qì* counterflow from engendering reversal.

B. Disease Patterns and Their Treatments in Summerheat Warmth Accompanied by Dampness

1. Summerheat-Damp Encumbering the Middle Burner

Pattern

Vigorous fever with vexation and thirst, copious sweating and scant urine, dilations in the stomach duct and subjective feeling of heavy body, and surging big pulse.

This pattern is characteristic of exuberant summerheat-heat at *yáng* brightness with a greater *yīn* damp obstruction. The symptoms of vigorous fever with vexation and thirst, copious sweating and scant urine, and surging big pulse are indicative of exuberant, formless pathogenic heat at *yáng* brightness. The symptoms of dilations in the stomach duct and subjective feeling of heavy body are indicative of a greater *yīn* damp obstruction.

Treatment

Clear *qì* and transform dampness.

Prescription

White Tiger Decoction Plus Atractylodes
(*Bái Hǔ Jiā Cāng Zhú Tāng* 白虎加蒼術湯)
From the *Book of Human Life* (*Huó Rén Shū* 活人書)

gypsum (*shí gāo*)	石膏	30g
anemarrhena [root] (*zhī mǔ*)	知母	12g
licorice [root] (*gān cǎo*)	甘草	3g
round-grained nonglutinous rice (*jīng mǐ*)	粳米	12g
atractylodes [root] (*cāng zhú*)	蒼術	10g

This pattern results from summerheat-damp encumbering the middle burner, but with *yáng* brightness summerheat-heat being primary, and greater *yīn* spleen dampness being secondary. White Tiger Decoction (*Bái Hǔ Tāng*) is therefore used to clear *yáng* brightness heat, and atractylodes [root] (*cāng zhú*) is added to transform greater *yīn* spleen dampness.

2. SUMMERHEAT-DAMP OVERFLOWING THROUGH THE TRIPLE BURNER

Pattern

Fever with red complexion and deafness, oppression in the chest and dilations in the stomach duct, congee-water-like stools, scant dark yellow urine, coughing of phlegm with blood in it, absence of severe thirst, red tongue, and slippery yellow moss.

This pattern is characteristic of summerheat-heat harboring damp and overflowing through the triple burner *qì* aspect. Since summerheat-heat steams outward there is fever that does not abate, and since it also steams upward to the head, face, and clear orifice there is also red complexion and deafness. As Yè Tiān Shì explained:

Dampness is a heavy turbid pathogen, and heat is a fuming steaming qì. When heat and dampness coalesce, the qì of immoderate steaming forces its way upward into the clear orifices and causes deafness, quite unlike that of lesser yáng deafness.

Lesser *yáng* deafness results from rising gallbladder heat, so it must be accompanied by alternating fevers and chills, bitter taste in the mouth, dry throat, and string-like pulse. Symptoms of damp-heat are therefore easily detected. When damp-heat overflows into the upper burner, heat detriments the lung network vessels and dampness obstructs the *qì* dynamic, so there is oppression in the chest and coughing of phlegm with blood in it. Summerheat-damp obstructs the middle burner, so there are dilations in the stomach duct and also an absence of severe thirst. Damp-heat brews and binds in the lower burner, so separation is impaired, the urine becomes scant and dark yellow, and the stools become congee-water-like.

This is different from heat bind circumfluence, where uninhibited congee-watery stool is always accompanied by abdominal tenderness. Red tongue and slippery yellow tongue moss are characteristic of pathogenic summerheat harboring damp in the *qì* aspect. Although this pattern can be ascribed to summerheat-damp, its pathomechanism involves the triple burner *qì* dynamic, so it is different from patterns where the pathomechanism exists in the middle burner spleen and stomach. In clinical practice, distinctions are easy to make.

Treatment

Clear heat and disinhibit dampness. Diffuse and throughclear the triple burner.

Prescription

Three Stones Decoction (*Sān Shí Tāng* 三石汤)

From the *Detailed Analysis of Warm Diseases* (*Wēn Bìng Tiáo Biàn* 溫病條辯)

Ingredient	Chinese	Dose
talcum (*fēi huá shí*) (ground in water)	飛滑石	10g
crude gypsum (*shēng shí gāo*)	生石膏	15g
glauberite (*hán shuĭ shí*)	寒水石	10g
apricot kernel (*xìng rén*)	杏仁	10g
bamboo shavings (*zhú rú*)	竹茹	6g
lonicera [flower] (*jīn yín huā*)	金銀花	10g
purified feces (*jīn zhī*)	金汁	10ml
rice-paper plant pith (*bái tōng căo*)	白通草	6g

Boil all the ingredients in five cups of water until two cups are left. Give while still warm, twice daily.

These symptoms are characteristic of heavy summerheat but light dampness. The disease site involves the *qì* aspect, but it is also located in the upper, middle, and lower triple burners. The treatment, therefore, must aim to clear and disinhibit triple burner damp-heat and to diffuse and throughclear the *qì* dynamic.

In Three Stones Decoction (*Sān Shí Tāng*):

§ Apricot kernel (*xìng rén*) is used to diffuse and open the upper burner lung *qì* so that when *qì* transforms, summerheat-damp transforms with it.

§ Crude gypsum (*shēng shí gāo*) and bamboo shavings (*zhú rú*) are used to clear and discharge middle burner pathogenic heat.

§ Talcum (*huá shí*), glauberite (*hán shuǐ shí*), and rice-paper plant pith (*tōng cǎo*) are used to clear and disinhibit lower burner damp-heat.

§ Lonicera [flower] (*jīn yín huā*) is used to flush summerheat and resolve toxins.

Since these are symptoms of heavy summerheat but light dampness, the principal medicinals in this prescription are used to clear summerheat and discharge heat, while the accompanying medicinals are used to disinhibit dampness.

3. SUMMERHEAT-DAMP ACCOMPANIED BY COLD

Pattern

Fever, aversion to cold, headache, absence of sweating, tetany, stomach duct oppression, vexation, and thin slimy tongue moss.

This pattern is characteristic of internal summerheat-damp with cold pathogens at the exterior. It usually occurs during the middle of summer, when pre-existing summerheat-damp conditions are compounded by intemperate living habits (e.g., sleeping in cool breezes or drinking cold drinks), and pathogenic cold traps summerheat-damp internally. Since cold fetters the exterior, defense *qì* is not throughclearing, the skin and body-hairs are blocked, and there are symptoms of fever, aversion to cold, headache, absence of sweating, and tetany. Moreover, since summerheat-damp is confined internally, there are also symptoms of vexation, stomach duct dilations, and slimy tongue moss. These symptoms result from simultaneous contraction of summerheat, dampness, and cold, with diseases of both the exterior and interior. They are quite different from the symptoms of isolated external wind-cold, and isolated *qì* damage from summerheat-heat.

Treatment

Course the exterior and scatter cold. Flush summerheat and transform dampness.

Prescription

Newly Supplemented Elsholtzia Beverage
(*Xīn Jiā Xiāng Rú Yǐn* 新加香薷飲)
From the *Detailed Analysis of Warm Diseases* (*Wēn Bìng Tiáo Biàn* 溫病條辯)

elsholtzia (*xiāng rú*)	香薷	6g
lonicera [flower] (*jīn yín huā*)	金銀花	10g
fresh lablab [bean] (*xiān biǎn dòu*)	鮮扁豆	10g
magnolia bark (*hòu pò*)	厚樸	6g
forsythia [fruit] (*lián qiào*)	連翹	6g

Boil all the ingredients in five cups of water until two cups are left. If sweating occurs discontinue medication; if sweating fails to occur continue medication.

Since there are symptoms of external cold and internal summerheat-damp occurring concurrently, the principal aim of treatment must be to resolve the exterior and scatter cold, whilst simultaneously flushing summerheat and transforming dampness.

Newly Supplemented Elsholtzia Beverage (*Xīn Jiā Xiāng Rú Yǐn*) is a variation of Three Agent Elsholtzia Powder (*Sān Wù Xiāng Rú Yǐn*). In it:

§ Elsholtzia (*xiāng rú*), which is acrid, warm, aromatic, and outthrusting, mainly courses the exterior and scatters cold but also flushes summerheat and transforms dampness.
§ Magnolia bark (*hòu pò*) dries dampness and harmonizes the middle [burner], rectifies *qì* and opens dilations.
§ Lonicera [flower] (*jīn yín huā*) and forsythia [fruit] (*lián qiào*) clear heat and flush summerheat.

The overall effect of this combination is to scatter cold, transform dampness, and flush summerheat.

C. ATTACHMENT: ENCROACHMENT OF SUMMERHEAT AND SUMMERHEAT FOULNESS

1. ENCROACHMENT OF SUMMERHEAT

Summertime common colds caused by summerheat-heat and damp pathogens, marked at onset by upper heater hand greater *yīn* lung channel symptoms, are called encroachment of summerheat.

Pattern

Chills and fevers with sweating, dizzy head, coughing, thin slightly slimy tongue moss, and floating pulse.

This pattern results from summerheat-heat and damp pathogens invading the upper burner lung defense. It is milder than summerheat warmth, its pathogenic tendency is comparatively shallow, and it normally has relatively fewer transmutations. Dizzy head and chills and fevers with sweating are characteristic of external summerheat pathogens. Coughing occurs when summerheat pathogens assail the lungs causing confinement that prevents diffusion to the exterior. Thin slightly slimy tongue moss results from mild summerheat-heat harboring damp. This pattern is called summerheat common cold, and is a type of summerheat disease in which the pathomechanism is not very serious.

Treatment

Clear and flush summerheat-heat while simultaneously disinhibiting dampness.

Prescription

Léi's Summerheat-Clearing, Cooling, and Flushing Method
(*Léi Shì Qīng Liáng Dí Shǔ Fǎ* 雷氏清涼滌暑法)

From the *Treatise on Seasonal Diseases* (*Shí Bìng Lùn* 時病論)

talcum (*huá shí*)	滑石	10g
raw licorice [root] (*shēng gān cǎo*)	生甘草	3g
rice-paper plant pith (*tōng cǎo*)	通草	3g
sweet wormwood (*qīng hāo*)	青蒿	5g
lablab [bean] (*bái biǎn dòu*)	白扁豆	3g
forsythia [fruit] (*lián qiào*)	連翹	10g
white poria (*bái fú líng*)	白伏苓	10g
watermelon rind (*xī guā cuì yī*) (use fresh)	西瓜翠衣	1pc

Boil all the ingredients in water.

These symptoms are characteristic of a mild summerheat upper burner disease, so a mild [heat] clearing prescription must be used to clear and outthrust the pathogenic heat.

In Léi's Summerheat-Clearing, Cooling, and Flushing Method:

- § Sweet wormwood (*qīng hāo*), lablab [bean] (*biǎn dòu*), forsythia [fruit] (*lián qiào*), and watermelon rind (*xī guā cuì yī*) clear and flush summerheat-heat and outthrust pathogens to the exterior.
- § Talcum (*huá shí*), licorice [root] (*gān cǎo*), and poria (*fú líng*) discharge heat and disinhibit dampness.

If there is also coughing, add apricot kernel (*xìng rén*) and trichosanthes rind (*guā lóu pí*) to diffuse the lungs and stop coughing.

2. SUMMERHEAT FOULNESS

When the *qì* of foul turbid summerheat-damp, contracted during the summer season, causes sudden oppression, vexation, and agitation, the disease is called summerheat foulness.

Pattern

Headaches with subjective sensations of distention, chest and stomach duct dilations and oppression, vexation and agitation, nausea and vomiting, skin heat with sweating, and in severe cases clouded spirit and deafness.

Summerheat foulness is usually referred to as "sand" and is a type of summerheat stroke that occurs between summer and autumn, when steaming summerheat-damp joins the foul turbid *qì* that is exuberant at that time, and intemperate lifestyles facilitate susceptibility to these pathogens. Summerheat-damp and foul turbidity associate and obstruct together—the *qì* dynamic is encumbered so there are chest and stomach duct dilations and oppression with vexation and agitation, and nausea and vomiting. Summerheat-damp is confined and steaming so there is sweating, but since the heat is not very strong the sweating is usually not profuse. Turbid damp *qì* obstructs the clear *yáng* so there are headaches with subjective sensations of distention. Moreover, in serious cases, turbidity can block the clear orifices and symptoms such as clouded spirit and deafness can result. This is different from heat falling into the pericardium where clouded spirit is accompanied by delirious speech, scorching heat and limb reversal, and crimson red tongue.

Treatment

Open the impurities and transform the turbidity with aroma.

Prescriptions

Agastache Qì-Righting Powder
(*Huò Xiāng Zhèng Qì Sǎn* 藿香正氣散)

From the *Imperial Grace Formulary* (*Hé Jì Jú Fāng* 和劑局方)

agastache (*huò xiāng*)	藿香	900g
perilla leaf (*sū yè*)	蘇葉	300g
angelica [root] (*bái zhǐ*)	白芷	300g
areca husk (*dà fù pí*)	大腹皮	300g
poria (*fú líng*)	茯苓	300g
ovate atractylodes [root] (*bái zhú*) (Stir-bake)	白術	600g
pinellia [tuber] leaven (*bàn xià qū*)	半夏曲	600g
tangerine peel (*chén pí*)	陳皮	600g
magnolia bark (*hòu pò*) (Prepare with ginger)	厚樸	600g
platycodon [root] (*jié gěng*)	桔梗	600g
honey-fried licorice [root] (*zhì gān cǎo*)	炙甘草	600g

Grind all the ingredients into powder and divide into 10-12g doses. Add two slices of ginger and one jujube (*dà zǎo*); boil in water, and administer. If sweating is imminent, cover the patient with cloths or blankets to encourage it.

Gate-Freeing Powder (*Tōng Guān Sǎn* 通關散)

From *Additions to the Teachings of Dān Xī* (*Dān Xī Xīn Fǎ Fù Yú* 丹溪心法附余)

small gleditsia [fruit] (*zhū yá zào*)	豬牙皂
asarum (*xì xīn*)	細辛

Grind equal quantities of both ingredients into powder and use as a snuff.

Jade Pivot Elixir (*Yù Shū Dān* 玉樞丹)
Also called Purple Gold Lozenge (*Zǐ Jīn Dìng* 紫金錠)

From *Book of Pure Heart Extracts* (*Piàn Yù Xīn Shū* 片玉心書)

musk (*shè xiāng*)	麝香	10g
shancigu [bulb] (*shān cí gū*)	山慈姑	100g
realgar (*xióng huáng*)	雄黃	30g
euphorbia/knoxia [root] (*dà jǐ*)	大戟	45g
caper spurge seed (*xù shuí zǐ*)	續隨子	30g
sumac gallnut (*wǔ bèi zǐ*)	五倍子	100g
cinnabar (*zhū shā*)	朱砂	30g

Grind all the ingredients except the musk (*shè xiāng*) into powder and blend thoroughly. Then mix in the musk with sticky-rice powder and water to form pills. Each pill should weigh about 10g. Take one pill, or in severe cases two pills per dose, and mix with cold water. This formula can also be purchased as a prepared medicine.

The key pathomechanism of this disease is summerheat-damp and foul turbidity confined and blocked at the interior. Therefore, Agastache Qì-Righting Powder (*Huò Xiāng Zhèng Qì Sǎn*) is used to repel the foul with aroma, rectify the *qì* and transform the dampness. If foul turbidity is clouding and blocking the clear orifices, use Gate-Freeing Powder (*Tōng Guān Sǎn*) as a nasal snuff to induce sneezing, and Jade Pivot Elixir (*Yù Shū Dān*) to repel the foulness with aroma and open the orifices.

CHAPTER 10
DAMP WARMTH

Damp warmth is an externally contracted hot disease that is caused by damp-heat pathogens, and therefore usually occurs during summer and autumn, when prevailing climates are rainy and humid. Its onset is relatively insidious, its transformations are relatively protracted, its disease impetus is lingering, its disease course is comparatively long, and it is marked by prominent spleen-stomach symptoms. Initially, there are clinical manifestations of unsurfaced fever, subjective sensations of heavy body and fatigued limbs, chest and stomach duct dilations and oppression, slimy tongue moss, and moderate pulse.

In clinical practice, damp warmth theory can be applied in pattern identification and treatment determination whenever biomedically defined conditions such as thyroid fever, paratyphoid fever, salmonella infection, acute schistosomiasis, leptospirosis, and influenza have prominent symptoms of dampness and smoldering heat.

I. DISEASE CAUSES AND PATHOLOGY

This disease is caused mainly by externally contracted damp-heat pathogens, but its ability to onset is closely related to the state of spleen and stomach functioning. Although it might occur at any time throughout the four seasons, it is generally seen during summer and autumn, when the weather is particularly rainy and humid—when celestial summerheat drives downward, earth dampness steams upward, and damp-heat is exuberant. The spleen and stomach are housed in the middle burner and govern transportation and transformation. If detriment and damage caused by dietary irregularities make it easy for dampness to collect and gather, or if the seasons of exuberant dampness, during which it is natural for spleen and stomach functionings to become comparatively tardy, make it easy for damp pathogens to encumber internally, external damp-heat pathogens readily invade the human body and the above disease can occur. As Xuē Shēng Bái explained:

> *When greater yīn is damaged internally, so that damp rheum collects and gathers, and guest pathogens arrive, internal and external interact with one-another causing damp-heat disease.*

This explains that damp warmth diseases usually engender because pathogens encumber both the interior and exterior simultaneously.

Due to the characteristic nature of their pathogens, the pathomechanic transformations and developments of damp warmth diseases are different from those of warm diseases in general. Dampness is a *yīn* pathogen with a heavy, turbid, slimy, stagnant nature. Thus, when it combines with heat it smolders and steams but does not transform—it becomes gluey, fixed, and difficult to resolve. Consequently, damp warmth diseases have relatively slower transformations than other warm diseases, their disease courses are comparatively long, and they are usually intractable.

Such diseases usually transmit from the exterior to the interior following a defense-*qì*-construction-blood progression. Initially, however, the core of disease transformation is in the middle burner spleen and stomach. The spleen is the damp-earth viscera and the stomach is the sea of water and food. So, when damp-heat causes disease, the core of disease transformation is usually in the spleen and stomach. As Zhāng Xū Gǔ wrote:

> *Since dampness corresponds with earth and the spleen corresponds with earth, they are linked by a single qì. Therefore, although damp-heat pathogens are initially contracted from the exterior, they later collect in the spleen and stomach.*

At the onset of this disease, pathogens contracted from the exterior encumber and trap the defense *yáng*, so there are transient symptoms of a defense aspect condition with accompanying symptoms of pathogenic dampness smoldering in the *qì* aspect of the spleen. There are, in short, both defense and *qì* aspect symptoms. As the external symptoms disperse, the *qì* aspect damp-heat slowly transmutes and grows exuberant. During this stage, dampness is trapped and heat is deep-lying, so smoldering and steaming are difficult to resolve, the cause is relatively obstinate, and the disease dynamic is relatively complex. Broadly speaking, dampness can be stronger than heat, heat can be stronger than dampness, or heat and dampness can both be strong. When dampness is stronger than heat the core of disease transformation inclines strongly to the spleen, and when heat is stronger than dampness the core of disease transformation inclines strongly to the stomach. As Zhāng Xū Gǔ comments:

> *Body yáng qì effulgence prompts speedy transformation to fire, which moves to yáng brightness; yáng qì vacuity prompts speedy transformation to dampness, which moves to greater yīn.*

This passage conveys that it is the nature of the human constitution that determines the relative strengths of dampness and heat. The stomach corresponds to *yáng* earth and governs dryness, and the spleen corresponds to *yīn* earth and governs dampness. Consequently, the nature of the human body is such that when *yáng* is effulgent, damp pathogens easily transform into dryness, heat becomes stronger than dampness, and the disease inclines to the stomach; when the *yáng* of the middle is insufficient, pathogens easily transform into dampness, dampness becomes stronger than heat, and the disease locates mostly in the spleen.

To trace the general development of damp warmth diseases, initially dampness contains smoldering heat, so there are usually manifestations of dampness stronger than heat, but as they develop, damp-heat slowly transforms into dryness, so there are manifestations of both strong dampness and heat, or even heat stronger than dampness. If damp-heat is confined and steaming in the *qì* aspect, despite the fact that the core of disease transformation is in the spleen or stomach, the disease pathogen can also spread through the triple burner, and by affecting the other bowels and viscera, can create numerous additional clinical manifestations. If damp-heat is confined and steaming externally under the skin, there can be miliaria alba; if it internally fumes the liver and gallbladder, there can be yellow jaundice; if it ascends and clouds the clear orifice there can be clouding of spirit knowledge; and if it descends and smolders in the bladder there can be inhibited urination.

Protracted damp-heat that smolders and steams without resolving at the exterior usually transforms into dryness and fire, so the pathomechanical transformations are more or less the same as those of general warm heat diseases. When in the *qì* aspect, heat causes symptoms of exuberant heat and damaged liquid (i.e., *yáng* brightness bowel repletion) and when in the construction-blood aspect, symptoms such as papules and macules, clouded spirit, reversal, and more often than not blood in the stools—because after dampness and heat have transformed into dryness and fire, they can easily damage the intestinal blood network vessels. Non-stop bleeding can lead to the dangerous consequence of *qì* deserting with the blood.

Provided this disease develops normally, during its final stage, the pathogenic heat gradually resolves but the human body remains weak. This is generally expressed in symptoms of right *qì* vacuity with adhering pathogens, or stomach *qì* under-arousal and spleen vacuity with failure of transporting function. After correct treatment, recovery normally ensues. On occasion, however, dampness remains encumbered; the *yáng qì* is detrimented and there are symptoms of kidney *yáng* vacuity and debilitation with retention of water dampness. As Yè Tiān Shì said, "When dampness prevails, *yáng* is debilitated."

II. MAIN POINTS OF DIAGNOSIS

1. During the initial stage of this disease, fever remains unsurfaced, but later as it gradually increases, there are persistently recurring weak fevers in the morning that grow stronger in the afternoons. Also, the head feels heavy as if bound, the body feels heavy and the limbs feel tired, there are feelings of oppression in the chest and dilations in the stomach duct, there is diarrhea or constipation, the tongue moss is slimy, and the pulse is moderate.

2. The transformations of this disease are relatively protracted, and the disease impetus is lingering. Damp-heat usually remains in the *qì* aspect for a comparatively long part of the disease course.

3. During the course of this disease not only miliaria alba, but also the serious symptom of passing blood from the bowels can occur. Moreover, during its final stage, if damp-heat transforms into dryness there can also be *yīn* damage, or if dampness prevails, *yáng* debilitation.

4. This disease most commonly occurs during the seasons of summer and autumn.

5. It is important that this disease be distinguished from summerheat warmth harboring damp. In summerheat warmth harboring damp there is exuberant *yáng* brightness summerheat-heat and accompanying greater *yīn* spleen dampness. Summerheat is the principal pathogenic *qì* and dampness is secondary. But in this disease dampness contains smoldering heat that steams and brews into warmth. Initially, dampness is principal—the heat pathogen is not very severe.

III. Pattern Identification and Treatment Determination

This disease develops from steaming and brewing of dampness that harbors smoldering heat. During its initial stage, dampness is usually stronger than heat, so the main aim of treatment must be to transform dampness. Depending on the symptom manifestations, use aromatic dampness transforming, bitter warm dampness-drying, and/or bland seepage-promoting dampness-disinhibiting methods to eliminate dampness and isolate heat.

Generally, at the beginning, internal and external pathogens combine, so dampness is trapped in both the defense and *qì* aspects. When this occurs, use a combination of aromatic dampness-transforming and diffusing-outthrusting methods to transform not only the exterior but also the interior dampness. After the exterior symptoms resolve, the main aim of treatment should be to diffuse and transform the *qì* aspect turbid damp pathogen and when necessary the secondary aim should be to clear the heat.

If, after the gradual transformation of dampness into heat, both dampness and heat become exuberant, use dampness-transforming and heat-clearing methods together. If after the damp pathogen transforms into heat, heat is stronger than dampness, treat principally by clearing heat and supplementarily by transforming dampness. If the dampness and heat have completely transformed into dryness and fire, administer treatments similar to those used for general warm diseases. If heat is intense in the *yáng* brightness *qì* aspect, treat by clearing heat and engendering liquid. If there is bowel repletion dry binding, treat by throughclearing the bowel and clearing the heat. When heat enters the construction-blood, and detriments and damages the intestinal passage and the blood network vessels so that blood passes with stools, treat by cooling the blood and stopping the bleeding. But if too much loss of blood leads to *qì* deserting with the blood, use emergency treatments to supplement the *qì* and stem its desertion.

After desertion returns and bleeding stops, use differential diagnosis and treatment to once again locate and restrain the underlying pathomechanism. During the recovery stage of this disease, if residual pathogens have not been cleansed and the *qì* dynamic is inhibited, give consideration to clearing and discharging the residual pathogens and to diffusing and disinhibiting the *qì* dynamic. If the disease pathogen has already resolved but the stomach *qì* is underaroused, or the transporting function of the spleen remains unfortified, use stomach-rousing and/or spleen-fortifying medicinals, according to the condition, to improve the prognosis. If, during the final stage, dampness that has remained encumbered for a prolonged period manifests a condition [that may be described as] "when dampness prevails, *yáng* is debilitated," and a transmuted pattern occurs, aim to warm the *yáng* and disinhibit the dampness.

A. DISEASE PATTERNS AND THEIR TREATMENTS IN DAMPNESS STRONGER THAN HEAT

1. PATHOGENS TRAPPED IN THE DEFENSE *QÌ*

Pattern

Aversion to cold with scant sweating, unsurfaced fever that gets stronger in the afternoons, heavy (feeling) head as if bound, subjective sensations of heavy body and fatigued limbs, oppression in the chest and stomach duct dilations, slimy white tongue moss, and soggy moderate pulse.

These symptoms are characteristic of dampness trapped in the defense and *qì* aspects with interacting of internal and external pathogens, and are usually seen during the initial stage of damp warmth. Aversion to cold with scant sweating is the manifestation of an external damp pathogen being confined and trapped in the defense *yáng*. Unsurfaced fever is the manifestation of dampness containing smoldering heat, or in other words, of heat-in-dampness. Since dampness and heat combine and steaming becomes more severe in the afternoon, fever gets stronger in the afternoon. Heavy [feeling] head as if bound occurs because the damp pathogen obstructs internally and prevents the clear *yáng* from upbearing. The subjective sensations of heavy body and fatigued limbs occur because dampness is lodging in the muscles and preventing the *qì* dynamic from diffusing. Oppression in the chest and stomach duct dilations occur because dampness is obstructing the *qì* aspect and preventing the *qì* from diffusing and being disinhibited. Slimy white tongue moss and soggy moderate pulse are both indicative of damp obstruction.

The symptoms of fever, aversion to cold, headache, and scant sweating are similar to cold damage external symptoms. However, in cold damage external symptoms, aversion to cold is comparatively strong, fever is comparatively insignificant, headaches and body pains are comparatively marked, there is absence of sweating, and the pulse is floating and tight. In this disease, aversion to cold and scant sweating are transient and of a lesser degree. Fever is unsurfaced, the head mainly feels clouded and distended (aching and pain are not marked), there are subjective sensations of cumbersome heavy body without much pain, the tongue moss is white, thick, and slimy, and the pulse is soggy and moderate rather than floating and tight. Moreover, there are concurrent symptoms of damp obstruction, like oppression in the chest and dilations in the stomach duct. These two patterns are therefore not very difficult to differentiate. In short, although this is the initial stage of the disease, there are not simply external symptoms, the disease is both external and internal; although this is a damp-heat disease, dampness is the principal pathogen—the heat pathogen is not very severe.

Treatment

Diffuse and transform with aroma.

Prescriptions

Agastache, Pinellia, and Poria Decoction (*Huò Pò Xià Líng Tāng* 藿樸夏苓湯)

From the *Principles of Medicine* (*Yī Yuán* 醫原)

agastache (*huò xiāng*)	藿香	6g
pinellia [tuber] (*bàn xià*)	半夏	5g
red poria (*chì fú líng*)	赤茯苓	10g
apricot kernel (*xìng rén*)	杏仁	10g
raw coix [seed] (*shēng yì rén*)	生薏仁	12g
nutmeg (*kòu rén*)	蔻仁	2g
polyporus (*zhū líng*)	豬苓	5g
alisma [tuber] (*zé xiè*)	澤瀉	5g
fermented soybean (*dàn dòu chǐ*)	淡豆豉	10g
magnolia bark (*hòu pò*)	厚樸	3g

Three Kernels Decoction (*Sān Rén Tāng* 三仁湯)

From the *Detailed Analysis of Warm Diseases* (*Wēn Bìng Tiáo Biàn* 溫病條辯)

apricot kernel (*xìng rén*)	杏仁	15g
talcum (ground in water) (*fēi huá shí*)	飛滑石	18g
rice-paper plant pith (*bái tōng cǎo*)	白通草	6g
cardamom (*bái kòu rén*)	白蔻仁	6g
bamboo leaf (*zhú yè*)	竹葉	6g
magnolia bark (*hòu pò*)	厚樸	6g
raw coix [seed] (*shēng yì rén*)	生薏仁	18g
pinellia [tuber] (*bàn xià*)	半夏	15g

Boil all the ingredients in eight cups of water until three cups are left. Give in one-cup doses three times per day.

Since these symptoms are characteristic of dampness trapped in the defense and *qì* aspects with interaction of internal and external pathogens, the most effective treatment is to dispel the external and internal dampness by diffusing and transforming with aroma.

In Agastache, Pinellia, and Poria Decoction (*Huò Pò Xià Líng Tāng*):

- Agastache (*huò xiāng*) and fermented soybean (*dàn dòu chǐ*) transform dampness at the exterior muscles by diffusing and outthrusting with aroma.

§ Apricot kernel (*xìng rén*) opens the lungs and disinhibits the *qì*, because when *qì* transforms it is easy for dampness to transform with it.

§ Magnolia bark (*hòu pò*), pinellia [tuber] (*bàn xià*), and nutmeg (*kòu rén*), promote transformation by drying dampness with warmth and bitterness.

§ Polyporus (*zhū líng*), red poria (*chì fú líng*), alisma [tuber] (*zé xiè*), and raw coix [seed] (*shēng yì rén*) disinhibit dampness by promoting seepage with blandness.

This formula resolves exterior and interior dampness, both externally and internally, by transforming dampness with aroma, drying dampness with warmth and bitterness, and disinhibiting dampness with bland seepage-promotion.

In Three Kernels Decoction (*Sān Rén Tāng*):

§ Apricot kernel (*xìng rén*) opens the lungs and disinhibits the *qì* to transform damp pathogens.

§ Cardamom (*bái kòu rén*), magnolia bark (*hòu pò*) and pinellia [tuber] (*bàn xià*) dry dampness and harmonize the center.

§ Rice-paper plant pith (*bái tōng cǎo*), raw coix [seed] (*shēng yì rén*), and talcum [ground in water] (*fēi huá shí*) mainly promote seepage with blandness and disinhibit dampness, but also discharge heat.

§ Bamboo leaf (*zhú yè*) assists in outthrusting heat.

When this formula is combined with Agastache, Pinellia, and Poria Decoction (*Huò Pò Xià Líng Tāng*), it helps to open above, diffuse the center, and percolate below. Agastache, Pinellia, and Poria Decoction contains agastache (*huò xiāng*) and fermented soybean (*dàn dòu chǐ*), which transform with aroma, outthrust, and discharge. Therefore it is best used for particularly strong external dampness. Three Kernels Decoction (*Sān Rén Tāng*) does not contain these medicinals but instead uses bamboo leaf (*zhú yè*) and talcum (*huá shí*), which discharge heat and disinhibit dampness. It is therefore more suitable when dampness contains smoldering heat.

During the beginning of this disease, sweat-inducing, attacking below, and *yīn*-enriching prescriptions are all contraindicated. If acrid warming sweat-inducing prescriptions are used erroneously, damp-heat can rise and cloud the clear orifice. If attacking-below prescriptions are used too early, the spleen and stomach *yáng qì* can be easily detrimented. And if *yīn*-enriching prescriptions are used, their slimy *yīn* softening natures can cause damp pathogens to stagnate, preventing them from transforming. As Wú Jú Tōng wrote:

> *Sweating clouds the spirit and deafens the ear, or in serious cases causes dimness of vision and loss of desire to talk; [attacking] below causes throughflux diarrhea; moistening prevents the disease from resolving.*

This passage describes the three contraindications that apply during the early stages of damp warmth diseases.

2. PATHOGENS IN THE MEMBRANE SOURCE

Pattern

Severe chills—slight fevers, body pain with sweating, subjective sensations of heavy hands and feet, vomiting with distention and fullness, thick white slimy turbid tongue moss, and moderate pulse.

These symptoms are characteristic of a particular type of damp-heat disease in which the pathomechanism is that severe turbid dampness confines and traps *yáng qì*. The symptoms of severe chills—slight fevers, body pain with sweating, and subjective sensations of heavy hands and feet are manifestations of a damp pathogen encumbering and trapping *yáng qì*, confining it and preventing it from extending to the exterior. They are not the same as symptoms caused by a cold damage cold pathogen fettering the exterior. Although the symptoms of cold damage include aversion to cold and body pain, they do not include sweating—the pathomechanism is completely different. Moreover, in this pattern there are accompanying symptoms of vomiting with distention and fullness, which are characteristic manifestations of internal obstruction by turbid dampness and unregulated *qì* dynamic. Thick white slimy turbid tongue moss and moderate pulse are both manifestations of internal obstruction by turbid dampness.

Treatment

Course, disinhibit, outthrust, and outpush.

Prescription

Léi's Membrane Source Diffusing and Outthrusting Method (*Léi Shì Xuān Tòu Mó Yuán Fǎ* 雷氏宣透膜原法)		
From the *Treatise on Seasonal Diseases* (*Shí Bìng Lùn* 時病論)		
magnolia bark (*hòu pò*) (prepare with ginger)	厚樸	3g
areca [nut] (*bīng láng*)	檳榔	5g
tsaoko [fruit] (*cǎo guǒ rén*) (roast in hot ashes)	草果仁	3g
scutellaria [root] (*huáng qín*) (stir-bake with wine)	黃芩	3g
shaved licorice [root] (*fěn gān cǎo*)	粉甘草	2g
agastache (*huò xiāng*)	藿香	3g
pinellia [tuber] (*bàn xià*) (prepare with ginger)	半夏	5g

Add three slices of fresh ginger (*shēng jiāng* 生姜) as an emissary.

This is a pattern in which turbid dampness is persistently severe and the pathological impetus is confining and blocking. Therefore, standard dampness-transforming methods are ineffective. Prescriptions that course, disinhibit, outthrust, and outpush must be used to open and outpush the turbid damp pathogens.

Léi's Membrane Source Diffusing and Outthrusting Method (*Léi Shì Xuān Tòu Mó Yuán Fǎ*) is a variation of Wú's Membrane Source Opening Beverage (*Wú Yòu Kě Dá Yuán Yǐn*). In it:

- § Magnolia bark (*hòu pò*), areca [nut] (*bīng láng*) and tsaoko [fruit] (*cǎo guǒ*) course and disinhibit turbid dampness.
- § Small quantities of scutellaria [root] (*huáng qín*) clear heat that is trapped and smoldering in dampness.
- § Licorice [root] (*gān cǎo*) harmonizes the middle.
- § Agastache (*huò xiāng*) and pinellia [tuber] (*bàn xià*) strengthen diffusing and transforming of turbid dampness.

Fresh ginger (*shēng jiāng*), which is acrid and outthrusting, is added to strengthen the outthrusting and outpushing function. This prescription is warming and drying, so it must not be used for longer than necessary. As soon as dampness opens and heat outthrusts, the heat impetus increases in severity, so the treatment method should be changed to clearing and transforming.

3. PATHOGENS IN THE MIDDLE BURNER

Pattern

Unsurfaced fever, dilations in the stomach duct and abdominal distention, nausea, absence of thirst or thirst with no desire to drink or thirst with liking for hot drinks, sloppy diarrhea, turbid urine, slimy white tongue moss, and soggy moderate pulse.

These symptoms are caused by a damp pathogen smoldering and obstructing the spleen and stomach. The disease is located in the middle burner, and the pathogenic impetus is provided by the strong damp pathogen. Dampness contains smoldering heat, so fever is unsurfaced. Dampness obstructs the *qì* aspect, so the clear *yáng* is unable to upbear and the head feels heavy, as if bound. Turbid dampness encumbers and obstructs the middle burner, so the *qì* dynamic is confined and there are dilations in the stomach duct and abdominal distention. The spleen and stomach lose control of the upbearing and downbearing functions, so turbid *qì* counterflows upward causing nausea, and the damp pathogen hastens downward causing diarrhea. Absence of thirst, or thirst with no desire to drink, or thirst with liking for hot drinks are characteristic of a damp pathogen obstructed internally. Slimy white tongue moss and soggy moderate pulse are characteristic of a strong damp pathogen.

Treatment

Dry dampness and transform turbidity.

Prescription

Léi's Aromatic Turbidity-Transforming Method
(*Léi Shì Fāng Xiāng Huà Zhuó Fǎ* 雷氏芳香化濁法)
From the *Treatise on Seasonal Diseases* (*Shí Bìng Lùn* 時病論)

agastache leaf (*huò xiāng yè*)	藿香葉	3g
eupatorium leaf (*pèi lán yè*)	佩蘭葉	3g
southern tangerine peel (*guǎng chén pí*)	廣陳皮	5g
processed pinellia [tuber] (*zhì bàn xià*)	制半夏	5g
areca husk (*dà fù pí*) (wash with wine)	大腹皮	3g
magnolia bark (*hòu pò*) (stir-bake with ginger juice)	厚樸	3g
fresh lotus leaf (*xiān hé yè*) (as an emissary)	鮮荷葉	10g

Since these symptoms are indicative of pathogens having entered the middle burner *qì* aspect, and are principally caused by strong damp pathogens, the main aim of treatment must be to dry dampness.

In Léi's Aromatic Turbidity-Transforming Method (*Léi Shì Fāng Xiāng Huà Zhuó Fǎ*):

§ Agastache (*huò xiāng*) and eupatorium leaf (*pèi lán*) transform dampness with aroma.

§ Tangerine peel (*chén pí*), pinellia [tuber] (*bàn xià*), areca husk (*dà fù pí*), and magnolia bark (*hòu pò*) dry dampness, rectify *qì*, and harmonize the middle.

§ Small quantities of fresh lotus leaf (*xiān hé yè*) assist in outthrusting and discharging pathogenic heat.

B. DISEASE PATTERNS AND THEIR TREATMENTS IN EQUALLY STRONG DAMPNESS AND HEAT

1. SMOLDERING DAMP-HEAT TOXINS

Pattern

Fever and thirst, dilations in the chest and abdominal distention, tired aching limbs, swollen throat and dark yellow urine, sometimes yellow body and eyes, and slimy yellow tongue moss.

These symptoms are characteristic of steaming dampness and heat confined and obstructed in the *qì* aspect with congestion of smoldering toxins above. Fever and thirst are manifestations of damp and heat steaming and rising. Dilations in the chest, abdominal distention, and tired aching limbs result from obstruction of smoldering damp pathogens encumbering the *qì* dynamic. Swollen throat is an expression of toxins congesting above, dark yellow urine is evidence of heat smoldering below, and slimy yellow tongue moss is a manifestation of equally exuberant dampness and heat. If steaming and obstructing of dampness and heat affect the gallbladder's coursing and discharging function, gallbladder fluids externalize so there will also be yellow body and eyes.

Treatment

Transform dampness and clear heat. Resolve toxins and disinhibit the throat.

Prescription

Sweet Dew Toxin-Dispersing Elixir
(*Gān Lù Xiāo Dú Dān* 甘露消毒丹)

From *Warm Heat Latitudes and Longitudes* (*Wēn Rè Jīng Wěi* 温热经纬)

talcum (*huá shí*)	滑石	450g
capillaris (*yīn chén*)	茵陳	330g
scutellaria [root] (*huáng qín*)	黃芩	300g
acorus [root] (*shí chāng pú*)	石菖蒲	180g
Sichuan fritillaria [bulb] (*chuān bèi mŭ*)	川貝母	150g
mutong [stem] (*mù tōng*)	木通	150g
agastache (*huò xiāng*)	藿香	120g
belamcanda [root] (*shè gān*)	射干	120g
forsythia [fruit] (*lián qiào*)	連翹	120g
mint (*bò hé*)	薄荷	120g
cardamom husk (*dòu kòu ké*)	豆蔻殼	120g

Sun-dry all the ingredients except the capillaris (*yīn chén*), and grind them into powder. Then boil the capillaris (*yīn chén*), mix its decoction with the powder to form small mung bean-sized pills, and coat these in medicated leaven (*shén qū*). Give 10g per dose with boiling water, or wrap 15-30g in gauze to be prepared as a decoction.

Since the functions of this prescription are to clear heat, disinhibit dampness, transform turbidity, and resolve toxins, it is commonly used for the treatment of damp warmth and summerheat-damp epidemics. In it:

- § Agastache (*huò xiāng*), cardamom husk (*dòu kòu ké*), and acorus [root] (*shí chāng pú*) are used to transform turbid dampness.
- § Scutellaria [root] (*huáng qín*) and forsythia [fruit] (*lián qiào*) are used to clear heat and resolve toxins.
- § Capillaris (*yīn chén*), talcum (*huá shí*), and mutong [stem] (*mù tōng*) are used to disinhibit dampness and clear heat.
- § Sichuan fritillaria [bulb] (*chuān bèi mŭ*) is used to disinhibit *qì* and scatter binding.
- § Belamcanda [root] (*shè gān*) is used to disinhibit the throat and disperse swelling.
- § Mint (*bò hé*) is used to assist by outthrusting and discharging pathogenic heat.

As soon as the dampness has been opened and the heat has been outthrust, the pathogenic impetus scatters and resolves.

2. DAMP-HEAT CONFINED AND OBSTRUCTED IN THE MIDDLE BURNER

Pattern

Fever accompanied but not resolved by sweating, thirst but little desire to drink, stomach duct dilations with nausea, vexation and oppression in the heart (i.e., the center of the chest), sloppy yellow stools, scant dark yellow urine, slimy yellow tongue moss, and slippery rapid pulse.

These symptoms are usually seen during the transformation of dampness into heat, when both dampness and heat are exuberant and steaming. Dampness is gradually transforming into heat, so internal heat is exuberant and there is fever that slowly increases. Damp-heat is steaming and rising so there is sweating. Heat is exuberant so there is thirst, but also damp pathogens are obstructed internally so even though there is thirst there is little desire to drink. Damp-heat is confined and steaming in the middle burner and the *qì* dynamic is obstructed and stagnant, so stomach duct dilations and nausea occur, together with vexation and oppression in the heart. Since damp-heat force-dries the intestinal passage, the lower heater loses its separating function, and there are sloppy stools with scant dark yellow urine. Slimy yellow tongue moss and slippery rapid pulse are characteristics of both dampness and heat exuberant.

Treatment

Transform dampness and clear heat.

Prescription

Wáng's Coptis and Magnolia Bark Beverage
(*Wáng Shì Lián Pò Yǐn* 王氏連樸飲)

From the *Treatise on Acute Disease with Vomiting and Diarrhea* (*Huò Luàn Lùn* 霍亂論)

Sichuan coptis [root] (*chuān lián*) (stir-bake in ginger juice)	川連	3g
processed magnolia bark (*zhì hòu pò*)	制厚樸	6g
acorus [root] (*shí chāng pú*)	石菖蒲	3g
processed pinellia [tuber] (*zhì bàn xià*)	制半夏	3g
fermented soybean (*dòu chǐ*)	淡豆豉	10g
stir-fried gardenia [fruit] (*chǎo shān zhī*)	炒山梔	10g
phragmites [root] (*lú gēn*)	蘆根	60g

Since the symptoms of this pattern are expressions of equally exuberant dampness and heat, treatment must be aimed not only at strongly clearing heat but also at strongly transforming dampness. Use Coptis and Magnolia Bark Beverage (*Lián Pò Yǐn*). In it:

- § Coptis [root] (*huáng lián*) and gardenia [fruit] (*shān zhī*), which are bitter cold medicinals, mainly clear heat but also dry dampness.
- § Magnolia bark (*hòu pò*) and pinellia [tuber] (*bàn xià*), which are bitter warm medicinals, dry dampness, downbear counterflow, and harmonize the stomach.
- § Acorus [root] (*shí chāng pú*) transforms impurities with aroma.
- § Fermented soybean (*dòu chǐ*) outthrusts and outpushes smoldering heat.
- § Phragmites [root] (*lú gēn*) mainly clears heat and disinhibits dampness but also engenders liquid.

When steaming of dampness and heat between the muscle and skin causes miliaria alba, add coix [seed] (*yì yǐ rén*) and bamboo leaf (*zhú yè*) to strengthen the dampness-seeping and heat-outthrusting functions.

3. DAMPNESS AND HEAT FERMENTING INTO PHLEGM AND CLOUDING THE PERICARDIUM

Pattern

Unabating fevers that are weaker in the mornings and stronger in the afternoons, spirit knowledge clouding (sometimes clear, sometimes hazy) or delirious speech, slimy yellow tongue moss, and soggy slippery rapid pulse.

These symptoms occur because damp-heat confined in the *qì* aspect steams without resolving, steaming ferments into turbid phlegm that clouds the pericardium, and the heart spirit loses control. Unabating fevers that are weaker in the mornings and stronger in the afternoons are characteristic of damp-heat smoldering and steaming in the *qì* aspect. Spirit knowledge clouding or delirious speech is an expression of damp-heat turbid phlegm clouding the pericardium—loss of agility by the orifice dynamic. Slimy yellow tongue moss and soggy slippery rapid pulse are reflections of damp-heat confined and steaming in the *qì* aspect. Although these symptoms can be attributed to pathogens invading the pericardium, they are also connected with internal clouding caused by brewing of damp-heat into turbid phlegm.

Internal blockage of the pericardium caused by heat entering the heart construction has somewhat different pathomechanics and treatments to this pattern. Its clinical manifestations include scorching heat with limb reversal, coma, non-stop mania with delirious speech or clouding with inability to speak, and crimson-red tongue. In clinical practice, these two patterns must be differentiated.

Treatment

Clear and disinhibit the damp-heat. Sweep the phlegm and open the orifices.

Prescriptions

Acorus and Curcuma Decoction (*Chāng Pú Yù Jīn Tāng* 菖蒲鬱金湯)

From the *Complete Compendium of Warm Disease* (*Wēn Bìng Quán Shū* 溫病全書)

fresh acorus [root] (*xiān shí chāng pú*)	鮮石菖蒲	3g
southern curcuma [tuber] (*guǎng yù jīn*)	廣鬱金	5g
stir-fried gardenia [fruit] (*chǎo shān zhī*)	炒山梔	6g
forsythia [fruit] (*lián qiào*)	連翹	10g
chrysanthemum [flower] (*jú huā*)	菊花	5g
talcum (*huá shí*) (wrapped in cloth)	滑石	12g
bamboo leaf (*zhú yè*)	竹葉	10g
moutan [root bark] (*dān pí*)	丹皮	6g
arctium [seed] (*niú bàng zǐ*)	牛蒡子	10g
dried bamboo sap (*zhú lì*) (add after decocting)	竹瀝	3 spoons
ginger juice (*jiāng zhī*) (add after decocting)	姜汁	6 drops
Jade Pivot Elixir (*Yù Shū Dān*) (add after decocting)	玉樞丹	2g

Imperial Grace Supreme Jewel Elixir (*Jú Fāng Zhì Bǎo Dān* 局方至寶丹)

From the *Detailed Analysis of Warm Diseases* (*Wēn Bìng Tiáo Biàn* 溫病條辯)

rhinoceros horn (*xī jiǎo*) (crushed)	犀角	30g
cinnabar (*zhū shā*) (water-ground)	朱砂	30g
amber (*hǔ pò*) (ground)	琥珀	30g
hawksbill [turtle] shell (*dài mào*) (crushed)	玳瑁	30g
bovine bezoar (*niú huáng*)	牛黄	12g
musk (*shè xiāng*)	麝香	15g

These days, use 90g of water buffalo horn (*shuǐ niú jiǎo*) instead of 30g of rhinoceros horn (*xī jiǎo*).

Liquid Storax Pill (*Sū Hé Xiāng Wán* 蘇合香丸)

From the *Imperial Grace Formulary* (*Hé Jì Jú Fāng* 和劑局方)

ovate atractylodes [root] (*bái zhú*)	白術	60g
valaimira (*qīng mù xiāng*)	青木香	60g
rhinoceros horn (*xī jiǎo*)	犀角	60g
cyperus [root] (*xiāng fù*)	香附	60g
cinnabar (*zhū shā*)	朱砂	60g
chebule (*hē lí lè*)	訶黎勒	60g
sandalwood (*tán xiāng*)	檀香	60g
benzoin (*ān xī xiāng*)	安息香	60g
aquilaria [wood] (*chén xiāng*)	沉香	60g
musk (*shè xiāng*)	麝香	60g
clove (*dīng xiāng*)	丁香	60g
long pepper (*bì bá*)	蓽拔	60g
borneol (*lóng nǎo*)	龍腦	30g
Liquid Storax Oil (*Sū Hé Xiāng Yóu*)	蘇合香油	30g
frankincense (*xūn lù xiāng*)	熏陸香	30g

These days, use 180g of water buffalo horn (*shuǐ niú jiǎo*) instead of 60g of rhinoceros horn (*xī jiǎo*). Grind all the ingredients except the Liquid Storax Oil (*Sū Hé Xiāng Yóu*) into powder and mix thoroughly. Then mix the Liquid Storax Oil with white honey, add the powder, and form pills.

Since this pattern occurs because damp-heat, which is confined and steaming in the *qì* aspect, ferments into phlegm and clouds the pericardium, it must be treated by clearing and disinhibiting damp-heat, sweeping phlegm, and opening the orifices. If heart-clearing orifice-opening prescriptions are used erroneously (because the spirit is clouded), cool is trapped and deep-lying "ice" is stored.

In Acorus and Curuma Decoction (*Chāng Pú Yù Jīn Tāng*):

- § Fresh acorus (*xiān chāng pú*) and curcuma [tuber] (*yù jīn*) diffuse the orifices with aroma.
- § Gardenia [fruit] (*shān zhī*), forsythia [fruit] (*lián qiào*), chrysanthemum [flower] (*jú huā*), moutan [root bark] (*dān pí*), arctium [seed] (*niú bàng zǐ*), and bamboo leaf (*zhú yè*) clear and discharge the heat pathogens.
- § Talcum (*huá shí*) scatters and disinhibits the damp pathogen.
- § Dried bamboo sap (*zhú lì*) clears and transforms phlegm-heat.

§ Ginger juice (*jiāng zhī*) and Jade Pivot Elixir (*Yù Shū Dān*) transform impurities and open blocks.

When used together, the overall effect of these medicinals is to clear heat and disinhibit dampness, transform phlegm and open the orifices. If there is an inclination towards stronger heat, use Supreme Jewel Elixir (*Zhì Bǎo Dān*). If turbid dampness is stronger, use Liquid Storax Pill (*Sū Hé Xiāng Wán*). If there are accompanying symptoms of stirring wind, such as convulsions, use Tetany Relieving Powder (*Zhǐ Jìng Sǎn*).

4. TURBID DAMPNESS CLOUDING ABOVE AND FAILURE OF SEPARATION

Pattern

Steaming heat with sensations of pressure in the head, vomiting and confounded spirit, urinary stoppage, thirst without much drinking, and slimy white tongue moss.

These symptoms result from damp-heat turbid pathogens encumbering and blocking the interior, clouding the clear orifices above, and obstructing the bladder below. Dampness traps heat, encumbering and obstructing the clear *yáng*, so there is steaming heat with sensations of distention in the head. Turbid pathogens invade the stomach, so the stomach loses its downbearing function and there is vomiting. Turbid dampness clouds the clear orifice above, so the spirit light loses clarity and the spirit clouds and confounds. Damp obstructions occur below and separation fails, so urinary stoppage ensues. Thirst without much drinking and slimy white tongue moss are characteristic manifestations of damp impurities obstructing internally.

Treatment

Begin by opening the orifices with aroma, and continue by promoting seepage with blandness, scattering, and disinhibiting.

Prescriptions

Liquid Storax Pill (*Sū Hé Xiāng Wán* 蘇合香丸)
From the *Imperial Grace Formulary* (*Hé Jì Jú Fāng* 和劑局方)

ovate atractylodes [root] (*bái zhú*)	白術	60g
valaimira (*qīng mù xiāng*)	青木香	60g
rhinoceros horn (*xī jiǎo*)	犀角	60g

cyperus [root] (*xiāng fù*)	香附	60g
cinnabar (*zhū shā*)	朱砂	60g
chebule (*hē lí lè*)	訶黎勒	60g
sandalwood (*tán xiāng*)	檀香	60g
benzoin (*ān xī xiāng*)	安息香	60g
aquilaria [wood] (*chén xiāng*)	沉香	60g
musk (*shè xiāng*)	麝香	60g
clove (*dīng xiāng*)	丁香	60g
long pepper (*bì bá*)	蓽拔	60g
borneol (*lóng nǎo*)	龍腦	30g
Liquid Storax Oil (*Sū Hé Xiāng Yóu*)	蘇合香油	30g
frankincense (*xūn lù xiāng*)	熏陸香	30g

These days, use 180g of water buffalo horn (*shuǐ niú jiǎo*) instead of 60g of rhinoceros horn (*xī jiǎo*). Grind all the ingredients except the Liquid Storax Oil (*Sū Hé Xiāng Yóu*) into powder and mix thoroughly. Then mix the oil with white honey, add the powder, and form pills.

Poria Skin Decoction (*Fú Líng Pí Tāng* 茯苓皮湯)

From the *Detailed Analysis of Warm Diseases* (*Wēn Bìng Tiáo Biàn* 溫病條辯)

poria skin (*fú líng pí*)	茯苓皮	15g
raw coix [seed] (*shēng yì rén*)	生薏仁	15g
polyporus (*zhū líng*)	豬苓	10g
areca husk (*dà fù pí*)	大腹皮	10g
rice-paper plant pith (*bái tōng cǎo*)	白通草	10g
bamboo leaf (*dàn zhú yè*)	淡竹葉	10g

Boil all the ingredients in eight cups of water until three cups remain, and give in three one-cup doses.

Since these symptoms result from damp-heat turbid pathogens causing internal obstructions and encumbering above and below, to start with, use emergency aromatic orifice-opening prescriptions that diffuse the orifice and rouse the spirit. Then later, add Poria Skin Decoction (*Fú Líng Pí Tāng*) to blandly promote seepage, scatter, and disinhibit. This throughclears and moves urine, to discharge turbid dampness below.

C. THE DISEASE PATTERN AND ITS TREATMENT IN HEAT STRONGER THAN DAMPNESS

Pattern

Unabating high fever, red complexion and rough breathing, thirst with desire to drink, subjective sensations of heavy body with dilations in the stomach duct, yellow slightly slimy tongue moss, and slippery rapid pulse.

This pattern is characteristic of dampness transforming into heat with heat stronger than dampness and the pathomechanism of exuberant heat in *yáng* brightness with smoldering dampness in greater *yīn*. The symptoms of high fever, vexation and thirst, red complexion and rough breathing are expressions of *yáng* brightness interior heat steaming and rising, while the subjective sensations of heavy body with dilations in the stomach duct are expressions of greater *yīn* spleen dampness. The yellow slightly slimy tongue moss and slippery rapid pulse are both indications that heat is stronger than dampness.

Treatment

Clear *qì* and transform dampness.

Prescription

White Tiger Decoction Plus Atractylodes
(*Bái Hǔ Jiā Cāng Zhú Tāng* 白虎加蒼術湯)
From the *Book of Human Life* (*Huó Rén Shū* 活人書)

gypsum (*shí gāo*)	石膏	30g
anemarrhena [root] (*zhī mǔ*)	知母	12g
licorice [root] (*gān cǎo*)	甘草	3g
round-grained nonglutinous rice (*jīng mǐ*)	粳米	12g
atractylodes [root] (*cāng zhú*)	蒼術	10g

Since these symptoms are due principally to exuberant *yáng* brightness heat, and secondarily to greater *yīn* spleen dampness failing to transform, use White Tiger Decoction Plus Atractylodes (*Bái Hǔ Jiā Cāng Zhú Tāng*) as the main remedy, to clear *qì* and discharge heat, and supplement with medicinals that transform greater *yīn* spleen dampness. If confined heat transforms into fire and damages the liquid, but not very seriously, add bitter cold medicinals such as coptis [root] (*huáng lián*) and scutellaria [root] (*huáng qín*).

D. THE DISEASE PATTERN AND ITS TREATMENT IN LINGERING RESIDUAL PATHOGENS

Pattern

Fever already abated, slight oppression in the stomach duct, hunger but no desire to eat, and slightly slimy tongue moss.

These symptoms can be seen during the recovery stage of a damp warmth disease. By this time the heat pathogens have already resolved; hence the fever has already abated, but there are still swirling clouds of residual pathogens. The *qì* dynamic is inhibited and the stomach *qì* is not soothed, so there is slight oppression in the stomach duct, hunger but no desire to eat, and slightly slimy tongue moss.

Treatment

Diffuse the *qì* and rouse the stomach. Clear and flush the residual pathogens.

Prescription

Xuē's Five-Leaf Phragmites Decoction
(*Xuē Shì Wǔ Yè Lú Gēn Tāng* 薛氏五葉蘆根湯)
From *Warm Heat Latitudes and Longitudes* (*Wēn Rè Jīng Wěi* 温热经纬)

agastache leaf (*huò xiāng yè*)	藿香葉	10g
mint leaf (*bò hé yè*)	薄荷葉	6g
fresh lotus leaf (*xiān hé yè*)	鮮荷葉	10g
loquat leaf (*pí pá yè*)	枇杷葉	10g
eupatorium leaf (*pèi lán yè*)	佩蘭葉	10g
phragmites [root] (*lú gēn*)	蘆根	12g
wax gourd seed (*dōng guā rén*)	冬瓜仁	12g

As Xuē Shēng Bái wrote:

When damp-heat has already resolved, but residual pathogens cloud the clear yáng and the stomach qì is not soothed, it is fitting that extremely light, clearing medicinals be used to diffuse the yáng-qì of the upper burner. Strong-flavored preparations should not be used.

This prescription contains:

- Five leaves, which lightly diffuse the *qì* dynamic and rouse the stomach with aroma.

§ Phragmites [root] (*lú gēn*) and wax gourd seed (*dōng guā rén*), which clear and disinhibit the residual damp-heat pathogens.

E. DISEASE PATTERNS AND THEIR TREATMENTS IN TRANSMUTED DAMP WARMTH

1. DAMP PATHOGENS TRANSFORMING INTO DRYNESS AND PASSING OF BLOOD WITH STOOLS

Pattern

Scorching heat with vexation and agitation, fresh blood passed with stools, and crimson-red tongue.

These symptoms result when damp-heat transforms into dryness and fire, enters deeply into the construction-blood, and forces blood to move below. Since in damp warmth the core of disease transformation is in the middle burner, as soon as pathogens transform into dryness they easily damage the intestinal blood network vessels, causing spillage of blood to occur below. Blood aspect heat toxins sear and intensify, so there are accompanying symptoms of scorching heat with vexation and agitation, and crimson-red tongue.

Treatment

Cool the blood and stop bleeding.

Prescription

Rhinoceros Horn and Rehmannia Decoction
(*Xī Jiǎo Dì Huáng Tāng* 犀角地黄湯)

From the *Detailed Analysis of Warm Diseases* (*Wēn Bìng Tiáo Biàn* 溫病條辯)

dried rehmannia [root] (*gān dì huáng*)	干地黄	30g
raw white peony [root] (*shēng bái sháo*)	生白芍	10g
moutan [root bark] (*dān pí*)	丹皮	10g
rhinoceros horn (*xī jiǎo*)	犀角	10g

These days, use 30g of water buffalo horn (*shuǐ niú jiǎo*) instead of 10g of rhinoceros horn (*xī jiǎo*). Boil all the ingredients in five cups of water until two cups are left. Give twice daily. Keep the remnants and use again.

Since the disease dynamic in this pattern is acute, treatments that cool the blood and stop bleeding must be administered immediately so that the bleeding can be quickly brought under control.

Rhinoceros Horn and Rehmannia Decoction (*Xī Jiǎo Dì Huáng Tāng*) is particularly good at cooling blood and resolving toxins, but in order to strengthen its anti-bleeding function, add supplements such as beauty-berry leaf (*zǐ zhū cǎo*), charred sanguisorba [root] (*dì yú tàn*), and charred biota leaf (*cè bǎi tàn*).

2. PASSING OF MUCH BLOOD WITH STOOLS; *YÁNG* VACUITY *QÌ* DESERTION

Pattern

Non-stop passing of blood with stools, pale complexion, sweating with cool limbs, dull lusterless tongue, and minute fine pulse.

This pattern is usually a one-step-further development of a disease in which a damp pathogen is transforming into dryness. Much blood is passed with the stools, so right *qì* deserts externally. The *qì* is the commander of the blood and the blood is the mother of the *qì*. Each is dependent on the other. Therefore, after sudden heavy loss of blood, since the *qì* has nothing to command, it promptly deserts and characteristic symptoms of *yáng* vacuity and *qì* desertion such as pale complexion, rapid loss of warmth, sweating with cool limbs, and minute fine pulse occur.

Treatment

Boost *qì* and stem desertion. Nourish blood and stop bleeding.

Prescriptions

Pure Ginseng Decoction (*Dú Shēn Tāng* 獨參湯)

From the *Divine Book of Ten Medicinal Agents* (*Shí Yào Shén Shū* 十藥神書).

ginseng (*rén shēn*)	人參	at least 60g

Yellow Earth Decoction (*Huáng Tǔ Tāng* 黃土湯)

From the *Synopsis of the Golden Chamber* (*Jīn Kuì Yào Luè* 金匱要略).

licorice [root] (*gān cǎo*)	甘草	90g
dried rehmannia [root] (*gān dì huáng*)	干地黄	90g
ovate atractylodes [root] (*bái zhú*)	白術	90g
aconite [accessory tuber] (*fù zǐ*) (stir-bake at high heat)	附子	90g
ass hide glue (*ē jiāo*)	阿膠	90g
scutellaria [root] (*huáng qín*)	黄芩	90g
oven earth (*zào zhōng huáng tǔ*)	灶中黃土	250g

In this pattern, the disease dynamic is critical so emergency measures must be taken to restore and boost the *qì* and to stem the desertion. Pure Ginseng Decoction (*Dú Shēn Tāng*) must be administered repeatedly until the symptoms of desertion have been stemmed, following which treatment must be prescribed according to condition. Once vacuity desertion has been brought under control, there is usually spleen and stomach vacuity and cold with *yīn* blood depletion and detriment. So most commonly, treatment must be aimed at warming and supplementing the spleen *yáng*, nourishing the blood and stopping the bleeding. Yellow Earth Decoction (*Huáng Tǔ Tāng*) contains:

§ Ovate atractylodes [root] (*bái zhú*), aconite [accessory tuber] (*fù zǐ*) and oven earth (*zào zhōng huáng tǔ*), which warm and supplement spleen *yáng*, astringe the intestines and stop bleeding.

§ Ass hide glue (*ē jiāo*) and raw rehmannia [root] (*shēng dì*), which nourish blood and stop bleeding.

§ Scutellaria [root] (*huáng qín*), which clears residual heat from the intestinal passage and counterbalances the acrid-hot natures of ovate atractylodes [root] (*bái zhú*) and aconite [accessory tuber] (*fù zǐ*).

§ Licorice [root] (*gān cǎo*) is added to harmonize the other ingredients. By applying cold and heat simultaneously, moisturizing and drying at the same time, this prescription attends to both *yīn* and *yáng* concurrently, warming the *yáng* without injuring the *yīn*—nourishing the *yīn* without detriment to the *yáng*.

3. PREVALENT DAMPNESS AND DEBILITATED *YÁNG*

Pattern

Physical cold and fatigued spirit, palpitations and dizzy head, swollen face and limbs, short voidings of scant urine, pale tongue with white moss, and sunken fine pulse.

These symptoms are the manifestation of a transmuted damp warmth pattern. They result when lingering damp pathogens damage the *yáng qì*, and are usually seen during the last stages of a damp warmth disease, where although the damp-heat has resolved, the *yáng qì* dynamic of the body has already been detrimented and damaged. As Yè Tiān Shì said, "Departure of damp-heat leaves *yáng* declining and debilitated." When the *yáng qì* is vacuous and declining, it is unable to warm and nourish the muscle interstices so there is physical cold with aversion to cold. The heart *yáng* is not roused so fatigued spirit and palpitations occur. Being vacuous, the *yáng* is unable to warm and transform water dampness so there are short voidings of scant urine, the head and eyes are dizzy, and the face and limbs are swollen. The pale tongue with white moss, and the sunken fine pulse are both manifestations of declining and debilitated *yáng qì*.

Treatment

Warm the *yáng* and disinhibit the water.

Prescription

True Warrior Decoction (*Zhēn Wǔ Tāng* 真武湯)

From the *Treatise on Cold Damage* (*Shāng Hán Lùn* 傷寒論)

poria (*fú líng*)	茯苓	90g
white peony [root] (*bái sháo*)	芍藥	90g
fresh ginger (*shēng jiāng*) (sliced)	生姜	90g
ovate atractylodes [root] (*bái zhú*)	白術	60g
aconite [accessory tuber] (*fù zǐ*) (stir-bake at high heat and cut into eight pieces)	附子	1 fruit

Since the pathomechanism of this pattern is declining and debilitated *yáng qì* with loss of warming and transforming function and consequential collecting of water-damp internally, it is treated with True Warrior Decoction (*Zhēn Wǔ Tāng*).

This prescription contains:

§ Poria (*fú líng*) and ovate atractylodes [root] (*bái zhú*), which boost *qì* and disinhibit water.

§ Fresh ginger (*shēng jiāng*) and aconite [accessory tuber] (*fù zǐ*), which warm *yáng* and scatter cold.

§ White peony [root] (*bái sháo*), which constrains *yīn* and harmonizes construction.

If there is prominent *qì* vacuity add codonopsis (*dǎng shēn*) to strengthen the *qì* supplementing function.

CHAPTER 11
LATENT SUMMERHEAT

Latent summerheat is an acute hot disease that occurs during autumn and winter and is marked by manifestations of summerheat-damp. Initially, there are characteristics similar to those of the common cold. Later, there are malaria-like symptoms, except that alternating fevers and chills lack periodicity. Later still there are symptoms of fever without aversion to cold that grows particularly strong at night and slightly decreased with sweating in the early morning, scorching heat in the chest and abdomen that does not eliminate, and diarrhea with unsatisfying defecation.

Its disease impetus is strong and therefore lingering, and because it occurs after summer, in either autumn or winter, it is often referred to as "late emergence," "latent summerheat autumn emergence," or "winter months latent summerheat." Different names are used according to different clinical manifestations. Latent summerheat theory can be applied in pattern identification and treatment determination for biomedically defined conditions such as influenza, leptospirosis, infectious encephalitis-B, and epidemic hemorrhagic fever.

I. DISEASE CAUSES AND PATHOLOGY

The outbreak of this disease can be attributed, initially, to contraction of a summerheat-damp disease pathogen, and then later to precipitation by an autumn or winter pathogen. Since summerheat-damp pathogens readily obstruct and trap the *qì* dynamic, outbreaks usually occur with pathogens in the *qì* aspect. But in people with *yīn* vacuous and *yáng* exuberant bodies, pathogens can easily transform into dryness and fire, and lodge in the construction aspect. Accordingly, pattern types differ depending on whether pathogens are in the *qì* or the construction aspect. Conditions are usually not severe when pathogens are in the *qì* aspect, but are severe when they are in the construction aspect. Severity is also influenced by another factor—by whether the disease appears earlier or later in the year. As Wú Jú Tōng commented:

> *When summerheat is contracted during long summer and appears after summer, its diseases are called latent summerheat. Diseases that appear before frost-fall are mild; diseases that do not appear until after frost-fall are more severe; diseases that appear during winter are most severe.*

No matter whether in the *qì* or construction aspect, this disease is always precipitated by seasonal pathogens. Therefore during its initial stage there are always accompanying defense aspect external patterns. After external pathogens that cause *qì* aspect patterns resolve, malaria-like clinical manifestations of summerheat-damp confined and steaming in lesser *yáng* are usually seen. If the disease transfers to the middle burner spleen and stomach before the damp pathogens have entirely disappeared, heat stronger than dampness patterns are usually seen; treatments similar to those for summerheat warmth with accompanying dampness and for damp warmth are given. As Wú Jú Tōng said:

> *Patterns of latent summerheat, summerheat warmth, and damp warmth all have the same source. These three diseases must be cross-referenced, without stubborn bias.*

Patients with internal accumulations and stagnations usually have summerheat-damp harboring stagnation. This manifests as diarrhea with unsatisfying defecation and scorching heat in the abdomen that does not eliminate. If the pathogen is in the construction aspect, the pathomechanisms, disease developments, patterns, and treatments are similar to those of other warm diseases with pathogens in the construction aspect.

II. MAIN POINTS OF DIAGNOSIS

1. This disease usually appears in autumn or winter.

2. This disease has a very rapid onset. As soon as it appears symptoms of summerheat-damp or latent summerheat internal heat occur. If it develops from the *qì* aspect there are symptoms of fever, vexation, thirst, dilations in the stomach duct, and slimy tongue moss; if it develops from the construction aspect there are symptoms of fever, dry mouth, vexation, and red tongue without moss. Initially, it is also accompanied by the external symptom of aversion to cold.

3. During the onset of this disease, the characteristics of summerheat-damp developing from the *qì* aspect are similar to those of common colds, but with accompanying internal summerheat-damp symptoms. Later however, pathogenic *qì* lodges at lesser *yáng* causing malaria-like alternating fevers and chills, but without periodicity. In clinical practice, distinctions should be made.

4. Occasionally during the course of this disease there are symptoms of fever without aversion to cold that grows particularly strong at night and slightly decreases with sweating in the early morning, scorching heat in the chest and abdomen that does not eliminate, and diarrhea with unsatisfying defecation. When these symptoms occur, damp-heat harboring stagnation and pathogenic heat confined in the intestines and stomach are indicated.

5. Damp-heat lingering in the *qì* aspect can cause miliaria alba, whereas if the pathogen lodges in the construction and heat forces its way towards the blood aspect there can be macules. Clinically therefore, diagnosis must be made according to systemic changes.

III. PATTERN IDENTIFICATION AND TREATMENT DETERMINATION

During the initial stages of this disease the exterior and interior are usually both affected together, so the primary aim of treatment must always be to resolve the exterior while simultaneously clearing the interior. But since internal patterns differ according to whether pathogens are in the *qì* or the construction aspect, this aim needs to be implemented flexibly. When *qì* aspect patterns occur with accompanying external patterns, [the treatment goal is to] resolve the exterior, clear the summerheat, and transform the dampness. When construction aspect patterns occur with accompanying external patterns, resolve the exterior and clear the construction. If external pathogens have already resolved, but summerheat-damp is confined to the lesser *yáng qì* aspect, clear and discharge the lesser *yáng*, scatter and disperse the damp-heat. If summerheat-damp harboring stagnation is confined to the intestinal bowel, use bitter acrid downward-throughclearing medicinals to course and throughclear the confined heat and dampness stagnation pathogens. If summerheat-damp transforms into dryness and enters the construction, so that pathogens cloud the pericardium, exuberant heat stirs blood, or liver wind stirs internally, patterns are usually similar to those seen in other warm diseases where pathogens enter the construction-blood aspect; therefore treat accordingly.

A. DISEASE PATTERNS OF BOTH THE EXTERIOR AND INTERIOR AND THEIR TREATMENTS

1. DEFENSE AND QÌ BOTH DISEASED

Pattern

Headache, whole body aches and pains, aversion to cold with fever, absence of sweating, vexation and thirst, scant dark yellow urine, stomach duct dilations, slimy tongue moss, and soggy rapid pulse.

These symptoms are characteristic of initial stage *qì* aspect latent summerheat with accompanying external symptoms. Headache, body ache, aversion to cold with fever, and absence of sweating are evidence of pathogens in the defense aspect. Vexation and thirst, and scant dark yellow urine are consequences of internally confined summerheat. Stomach duct dilations and slimy tongue moss are the result of damp pathogens obstructing the *qì* aspect. Soggy rapid pulse occurs because dampness is confined and heat is steaming. These manifestations are similar to those of cold damage caused by autumn and winter external wind-cold, and those of common colds. Initially, all have defense aspect external symptoms, but their patterns and conditions are different, so they must not be confused. In external wind-cold, there are only ever manifestations of aversion to cold with fever, headache, and absence of sweating. There are never manifestations of internally confined summerheat-damp such as thirst and slimy tongue moss. In this pattern, there are both external and internal manifestations.

Treatment

Resolve the exterior, clear the summerheat, and transform the dampness. Lonicera and Forsythia Powder (*Yín Qiào Săn* 銀翹散) or Coptis [Root] and Elsholtzia Beverage (*Huáng Lián Xiāng Rú Yĭn* 黃連香薷飲) may be used according to the condition.

Prescriptions

Lonicera and Forsythia Powder (*Yín Qiào Săn* 銀翹散)
Plus apricot kernel (*xìng rén* 杏仁), talcum (*huá shí* 滑石), coix [seed] (*yì yĭ rén* 意苡仁) and rice-paper plant pith (*tōng căo* 通草)
From the *Detailed Analysis of Warm Diseases* (*Wēn Bìng Tiáo Biàn* 溫病條辯)

lonicera [flower] (*jīn yín huā*)	金銀花	10g
forsythia [fruit] (*lián qiào*)	連翹	10g
platycodon [root] (*jié gĕng*)	桔梗	6g
arctium [seed] (*niú bàng zĭ*) (crush)	牛蒡子	10g
mint (*bò hé*) (add later)	薄荷	6g
fermented soybean (*dòu chĭ*)	淡豆豉	10g
schizonepeta (*jīng jiè*)	荆芥	12g
bamboo leaf (*dàn zhú yè*)	淡竹葉	10g
fresh phragmites [root] (*xiān lú gēn*)	鮮蘆根	10g
raw licorice [root] (*shēng gān căo*)	生甘草	6g
northern apricot kernel (*bĕi xìng rén*)	北杏仁	10g
talcum (*huá shí*) (wrap in cloth)	滑石	20g
coix [seed] (*yì yĭ rén*)	意苡仁	12g
rice-paper plant pith (*tōng căo*)	通草	10g

Coptis [Root] and Elsholtzia Beverage (*Huáng Lián Xiāng Rú Yĭn* 黃連香薷飲)
From *Commentary on the Book of Human Life* (*Lèi Zhèng Huó Rén Shū* 類證活人書)

elsholtzia (*xiāng rú*)	香薷	10g
lablab [bean] (*biăn dòu*)	扁豆	12g
magnolia bark (*hòu pò*)	厚樸	10g
coptis [root] (*huáng lián*)	黃連	6g

Externally there are exterior pathogens that require acrid scattering exterior-resolving treatments; internally there is summerheat-damp that requires heat-clearing dampness-transforming treatments. Thus Lonicera and Forsythia Powder (*Yín Qiào Săn*) is prescribed to acridly cool, course, and resolve the defense aspect pathogens. Apricot kernel (*xìng rén*), talcum (*huá shí*), coix [seed] (*yì yĭ rén*), and rice-paper plant pith (*tōng căo*) are added to clear and disinhibit the summerheat-damp from the interior. Since the lungs govern the *qì* of the entire body, and when *qì* transforms it is easy for dampness to transform with it, apricot kernel (*xìng rén*) is used to open the lungs and disinhibit the *qì*. Talcum (*huá shí*), which is sweet and bland, is used to clear and disinhibit the summerheat-damp pathogens. Coix [seed] (*yì yĭ rén*) and rice-paper plant pith (*tōng căo*), which are both bland, are used to promote seepage and disinhibit dampness.

In combination, these medicinals resolve both the external and internal pathogens. If the internal dampness transforms into heat, which causes vexation and more severe thirst, use Coptis [Root] and Elsholtzia Beverage (*Huáng Lián Xiāng Rú Yĭn*). This prescription is also called Four Agents Elsholtzia Decoction (*Sì Wù Xiāng Rú Yĭn*). It consists of elsholtzia (*xiāng rú*), magnolia bark (*hòu pò*), and lablab [bean] (*biăn dòu*), which resolve the exterior and scatter cold, flush summerheat and transform dampness, plus coptis [root] (*huáng lián*), which clears heart heat and eliminates vexation.

2. DEFENSE AND CONSTRUCTION BOTH DISEASED

Pattern

Fever with slight aversion to cold, headache, scant sweating, dry mouth without thirst, vexation, red tongue with scant moss, and floating fine rapid pulse.

This pattern is characteristic of latent summerheat developing from the construction aspect with accompanying external symptoms. External pathogens assail the exterior so fever with aversion to cold, headache, and scant sweating develops. Summerheat-heat transforms into dryness and heat lodges in the construction aspect so there are symptoms of vexation and red tongue with scant moss. The pulses are floating, fine, and rapid because the construction *yīn* is insufficient and there are accompanying exterior patterns.

This pattern must be differentiated from the immediately preceding pattern. Both patterns are caused by latent summerheat, and initially both appear with symptoms of diseased exterior and interior. But internal heat lodging in the *qì* has differences from internal heat lodging in the construction, and there are also differences between summerheat-damp confined and steaming and summerheat-damp transforming into dryness. So, although the external pattern remains the same, different internal patterns are seen. In diseases of both defense and *qì*, summerheat-damp is confined to the *qì* aspect, so there are symptoms of thirst, slimy tongue moss, and soggy rapid pulse. In this pattern, summerheat-damp transforms into dryness and pathogens lodge in the construction aspect, so there are symptoms of dry mouth without thirst, red tongue with scant moss, and floating fine rapid pulse.

Treatment

Resolve the exterior and clear the construction.

Prescription

Lonicera and Forsythia Powder (*Yín Qiào Săn* 銀翹散)

Plus raw rehmannia [root] (*shēng dì* 生地), moutan [root bark] (*dān pí* 丹皮), red peony [root] (*chì sháo* 赤芍), and ophiopogon [tuber] (*mài dōng* 麥冬).

From the *Detailed Analysis of Warm Diseases* (*Wēn Bìng Tiáo Biàn* 溫病條辯)

lonicera [flower] (*jīn yín huā*)	金銀花	10g
forsythia [fruit] (*lián qiào*)	連翹	10g
platycodon [root] (*jié gěng*)	桔梗	6g
arctium [seed] (*niú bàng zǐ*) (crush)	牛蒡子	10g
mint (*bò hé*) (add later)	薄荷	6g
fermented soybean (*dòu chǐ*)	淡豆豉	10g
schizonepeta (*jīng jiè*)	荊芥	12g
bamboo leaf (*dàn zhú yè*)	淡竹葉	10g
fresh phragmites [root] (*xiān lú gēn*)	鮮蘆根	10g
raw licorice [root] (*shēng gān căo*)	生甘草	6g
raw rehmannia [root] (*shēng dì*)	生地	15g
moutan [root bark] (*dān pí*)	丹皮	10g
red peony [root] (*chì sháo*)	赤芍	10g
ophiopogon [tuber] (*mài dōng*)	麥冬	10g

One of the factors to which this pattern can be attributed is external pathogens at the exterior, so Lonicera and Forsythia Powder (*Yín Qiào Săn*), an acrid cool exterior-resolving prescription, is used to course and resolve defense aspect pathogens. The other factor is internal heat in the construction aspect. To address this, moutan [root bark] (*dān pí*) and red peony [root] (*chì sháo*) are added to cool construction and discharge heat, along with raw rehmannia [root] (*shēng dì*) and ophiopogon [tuber] (*mài dōng*) to clear construction and enrich liquid.

B. DISEASE PATTERNS AND THEIR TREATMENTS IN PATHOGENS IN THE *QÌ* ASPECT

1. PATHOGENS IN LESSER *YÁNG*

Pattern

Malaria-like alternating fevers and chills, thirst and vexation, stomach duct dilations, fever increasing during the afternoon that grows particularly strong at night and becomes slightly decreased with sweating in the early morning, scorching heat in the chest and abdomen that does not eliminate, slimy yellow-white tongue moss, and string-like rapid pulse.

These symptoms occur when summerheat-damp pathogens are confined in the lesser *yáng qì* aspect. The lesser *yáng* gate-mechanism is inhibited, so there are malaria-like alternating fevers and chills, and a string-like rapid pulse. Summerheat-heat is steaming internally, so there is vexation and thirst. Damp pathogens are obstructed internally, so there are stomach duct dilations and the tongue moss is slimy. During the late afternoon the battle between summerheat and dampness intensifies, so fever increases and grows particularly strong at night. Distressful steaming of summerheat-heat discharges externally, so even though damp pathogens are obstructed, slight sweating occurs during the early morning and the whole pattern eases slightly—except for the scorching heat in the chest and abdomen, which does not eliminate. This pattern must be differentiated from malaria. In malaria, all symptoms temporarily disappear after sweating and reappear periodically. But in this pattern there is no periodicity.

Treatment

Clear and discharge lesser *yáng*.

Prescriptions

Sweet Wormwood and Scutellaria Gallbladder-Clearing Decoction (*Hāo Qín Qīng Dǎn Tāng* 蒿芩清膽湯)

From the *Popularized Treatise on Cold Damage* (*Tōng Sú Shāng Hán Lùn* 通俗傷寒論)

sweet wormwood (*qīng hāo*)	青蒿	5-6g
scutellaria [root] (*huáng qín*)	黃芩	5-10g
bamboo shavings (*dàn zhú rú*)	淡竹茹	10g
pinellia [tuber] (*bàn xià*)	半夏	5g
bitter orange (*zhǐ qiào*)	枳殼	4g
tangerine peel (*chén pí*)	陳皮	5g
red poria (*chì fú líng*)	赤茯苓	10g
Jasper Jade Powder (*Bì Yù Sǎn*) (wrap in cloth)	碧玉散	10g

The lesser *yáng* gate-mechanism is inhibited; gallbladder heat is intense and exuberant, and summerheat-heat is confined internally.

In this formula:

§ Sweet wormwood (*qīng hāo*) and scutellaria [root] (*huáng qín*) are used to clear and discharge the lesser *yáng* gallbladder heat and to disinhibit the gate-mechanism.

§ Pinellia [tuber] (*bàn xià*), tangerine peel (*chén pí*), bitter orange (*zhǐ qiào*), and bamboo shavings (*dàn zhú rú*) are used to rectify the *qì*, harmonize the stomach, and transform the dampness.

§ Red poria (*chì fú líng*) and Jasper Jade Powder (*Bì Yù Sǎn*) are used to clear and disinhibit the damp-heat.

2. PATHOGENS BINDING IN THE INTESTINAL BOWEL

Pattern

Scorching heat in the chest and abdomen, nausea and vomiting, yellow-ochre colored diarrhea with unsatisfying defecation, slimy yellow grimy tongue moss, and soggy rapid pulse.

These symptoms are characteristic of summerheat-damp confined and steaming in the *qì* aspect with accompanying food stagnation. Summerheat-damp accumulations and stagnations obstruct the intestinal passageway, so there is noxious-smelling yellow-ochre colored diarrhea with unsatisfying defecation. The stomach *qì* loses its downbearing function and counterflows upward, so there is nausea and vomiting. Damp-heat is confined and steaming internally, so there is scorching heat in the chest and abdomen. The slimy yellow tongue moss and the soggy rapid pulse are indications of internal damp-heat. Both this pattern and the immediately preceding pattern are caused by pathogens in the *qì* aspect, but each has a different core of disease transformation. In the immediately preceding pattern the core of disease transformation is in the lesser *yáng*, whereas in this pattern the core of disease transformation is in the intestinal passageway.

Treatment

Abduct stagnation and throughclear below. Clear heat and transform dampness.

Prescriptions

Unripe Bitter Orange Stagnation-Abducting Decoction
(*Zhǐ Shí Dǎo Zhì Tāng* 枳實導滯湯)

From the *Popularized Treatise on Cold Damage* (*Tōng Sú Shāng Hán Lùn* 通俗傷寒論).

unripe bitter orange (*zhǐ shí*)	枳實	6g
raw rhubarb (*shēng dà huáng*) (wash with wine)	生大黃	5g
crataegus [fruit] (*shān zhā*)	山楂	10g
areca [nut] (*bīng láng*)	檳榔	5g
Sichuan magnolia bark (*chuān hòu pò*)	川厚樸	5g
Sichuan coptis [root] (*chuān huáng lián*)	川黃連	2g
Six Ingredient Leaven (*liù qū*)	六曲	10g
forsythia [fruit] (*lián qiào*)	連翹	5g
puccoon (*zǐ cǎo*)	紫草	10g
mutong [stem] (*mù tōng*)	木通	4g
licorice [root] (*gān cǎo*)	甘草	2g

Since in this pattern pathogens stagnate in the intestinal passageway, results cannot be achieved without attacking below. Furthermore, since summerheat-damp is confined internally, it is also necessary to clear and transform. Unripe Bitter Orange Stagnation-Abducting Decoction (*Zhǐ Shí Dǎo Zhì Tāng*) is therefore used not only for its bitter acrid downward-throughclearing action, but also for its ability to transform damp-heat accumulations and stagnations. In this formula:

§ Rhubarb (*shēng dà huáng*), unripe bitter orange (*zhǐ shí*), magnolia bark (*hòu pò*), and areca [nut] (*bīng láng*) not only push and flush accumulations and stagnation, but also rectify *qì*, transform dampness, and discharge heat.

§ Crataegus [fruit] (*shān zhā*) and Six Ingredient Leaven (*liù qū*) disperse, abduct, and harmonize the middle.

§ Coptis [root] (*huáng lián*), forsythia [fruit] (*lián qiào*), and puccoon (*zǐ cǎo*) clear heat and resolve toxins.

§ Mutong [stem] (*mù tōng*) disinhibits dampness and clears heat.

§ Licorice [root] (*gān cǎo*) harmonizes the other ingredients.

Since in this pattern damp-heat accumulations and stagnations adhere to and stagnate in the intestinal passageways, disease pathogens are not removed the first time a prescription is used to attack below. The attacking-below method generally needs to be used over and over again. Consequently, mild preparations are appropriate; strong preparations are inappropriate. Clinically, when the above case is seen, the signs of heat reappear shortly after each bowel movement, and there is diarrhea with unsatisfying defecation. Therefore, the attacking below method must be used to abduct and move heat downward, until the damp-heat stagnation pathogen has dispersed. As Yè Tiān Shì said:

> *When cold damage pathogenic heat existing at the interior robs and scorches the fluids, the appropriate treatment is to strongly [attack] below. But here, the main problem is that damp pathogens fight internally, so the appropriate treatment is to mildly [attack] below. In cold damage diseases diarrhea means that the pathogens are already finished so it is inappropriate to continue [attacking] below, but in damp warmth diseases, diarrhea means that the pathogens are not yet finished. It is only when the stools are hard that care must be taken not to continue attacking. When the stools are dry it means that there is no longer any dampness.*

C. DISEASE PATTERNS AND THEIR TREATMENTS IN PATHOGENS IN THE CONSTRUCTION-BLOOD ASPECT

1. HEAT IN THE HEART CONSTRUCTION TRANSFERRING DOWNWARD TO THE SMALL INTESTINES

Pattern

Fever that is mild during the day but severe at night, vexation and insomnia, dry mouth, thirst but no desire to drink, scant dark yellow urine that causes burning pain when passed, and crimson tongue.

These symptoms are characteristic of heat in the heart construction transferring downward to the small intestines. Fever that grows more severe at night, dry mouth, and crimson tongue are evidence that scorching summerheat-heat has entered the construction, and that the *yīn* construction has been detrimented. Vexation and insomnia are expressions of the heart spirit being harassed by heat. The heart and small intestines have an interior-exterior relationship, so when heart construction heat pathogens transfer downward to the small intestines, they manifest as the accompanying symptom of scant dark yellow urine that causes burning pain when passed (the main characteristic of small intestine exuberant heat). This is a pattern in which the heart construction and small intestines are both diseased, so it is not the same as a simple pattern of intense heart construction heat. The key difference is that in this pattern there is accompanying bowel fire exuberant heat.

Treatment

Clear the heart and cool construction. Clear and drain bowel fire.

Prescriptions

Red-Abducting Heart-Clearing Decoction
(*Dǎo Chì Qīng Xīn Tāng* 導赤清心湯)

From the *Popularized Treatise on Cold Damage* (*Tōng Sú Shāng Hán Lùn* 通俗傷寒論).

fresh raw rehmannia [root] (*xiān shēng dì*)	鮮生地	20g
cinnabar [coated] root poria (*zhū fú shén*)	朱茯神	6g
thin mutong [stem] (*xì mù tōng*)	細木通	2g
crude ophiopogon [tuber] (*yuán mài dōng*) (dyed with cinnabar)	原麥冬	3g
powdered moutan [root bark] (*fěn dān pí*)	粉丹皮	6g
Origin-Boosting Powder (*Yì Yuán Sǎn*) (wrap in cloth)	益元散	10g
bamboo leaf (*dàn zhú yè*)	淡竹葉	5g
lotus embryo (*lián zǐ xīn*)	連子心	30 kernels
juncus [pith] (*dēng xīn cǎo*) (dyed with cinnabar)	燈心草	20pc
child's urine (*tóng biàn*)	童便	1 glass

Since this pattern results from heat in the heart construction it must be treated by clearing the heart and cooling the construction, but since there is also exuberant small intestine heat it is essential to clear and drain bowel fire. Red-Abducting Heart-Clearing Decoction (*Dǎo Chì Qīng Xīn Tāng*) is ideally suited to these ends. In it:

- Raw rehmannia [root] (*shēng dì*), ophiopogon [tuber] (*mài dōng*), and moutan [root bark] (*dān pí*) clear construction (heat) and enrich humor.

§ Root poria (*fú shén*), lotus embryo (*lián zǐ xīn*), and juncus [pith] (*dēng xīn cǎo*) dyed with cinnabar clear heart heat to quiet the heart spirit.

§ Mutong [stem] (*mù tōng*), bamboo leaf (*zhú yè*), Origin-Boosting Powder (*Yì Yuán Sǎn*), and child's urine (*tóng biàn*) clear and abduct small intestine heat.

As soon as the heart construction has been cleared of heat, small intestine heat resolves and all the associated symptoms disperse. Therefore, as can be seen, the name of this formula is taken from its functions. Since it is made from Red-Abducting Powder (*Dǎo Chì Sǎn*) plus ophiopogon [tuber] (*mài dōng*), lotus embryo (*lián xīn*), moutan [root bark] (*dān pí*), and root poria (*fú shén*), it is better than Red-Abducting Powder at clearing construction [heat], nourishing humor, and quieting the spirit.

2. HEAT BLOCK IN THE PERICARDIUM; BLOOD NETWORK VESSEL STASIS

Pattern

Fever that grows stronger at night, clouded spirit and delirious speech, desire to rinse [the mouth] with water but aversion to getting the throat wet, crimson tongue without moss that looks dry but feels moist to the touch or looks dark-purple and moist.

These symptoms are characteristic of heat block in the pericardium with blood network vessel stasis. Fever grows stronger at night because heat is in the construction [aspect]. Clouded spirit and delirious speech occur because there is a pathogen block in the pericardium. Crimson tongue that looks dry but feels moist to the touch or looks purple and moist, is not a symptom of desiccated fluids, but of blood stasis. Desire to rinse [the mouth] with water but aversion to getting the throat wet, or dry mouth but no desire to drink, are characteristic of blood network vessel stasis. This and the immediately preceding pattern both result from heat in the heart construction. But the immediately preceding pattern is accompanied by exuberant small intestine heat, whereas this pattern is marked by a pathogen block in the pericardium with blood network vessel stasis. Therefore, both have different clinical manifestations.

Treatment

Clear the construction and discharge heat. Open the orifices and throughclear stasis.

Prescriptions

Rhinoceros Horn and Rehmannia Network-Quickening Beverage (*Xī Dì Qīng Luò Yǐn* 犀地清絡飲)

From the *Popularized Treatise on Cold Damage* (*Tōng Sú Shāng Hán Lùn* 通俗傷寒論).

rhinoceros horn juice (*xī jiǎo zhī*) (mixed with water)	犀角汁	4 spoons
powdered moutan [root bark] (*fěn dān pí*)	粉丹皮	6g
unripe forsythia [fruit] (*qīng lián qiào*) (uncored)	青連翹	5g
dried bamboo sap (*dàn zhú lì*) (stirred)	淡竹瀝	10 spoons
fresh raw rehmannia [root] (*xiān shēng dì*)	鮮生地	25g
raw red peony [root] (*shēng chì sháo*)	生赤芍	5g
unhusked peach kernel (*yuán táo rén*)	原桃仁	9 kernels
raw ginger juice (*shēng jiāng zhī*) (mixed with water)	生姜汁	2 drops

These days, use water buffalo horn (*shuǐ niú jiǎo*) instead of rhinoceros horn (*xī jiǎo*). Take 30g of fresh imperata [root] (*xiān máo gēn*) and five juncus roots (*dēng xīn gēn*); simmer them in water. Remove the residue and use the remaining fluid to decoct the other medicinals. Give with two tablespoons of fresh acorus [root] juice (*xiān shí chāng pǔ zhī*).

This pattern reflects intense heat in the construction, and so must be treated by clearing the construction and discharging heat. But because there are accompanying symptoms of a pathogen block in the pericardium, medicinals that clear the heart and open the orifices must be added, and because there are also accompanying symptoms of blood network vessel stasis, medicinals that quicken the blood and throughclear the stasis must be added as well. Treatment must aim not only to clear the construction and discharge heat, but also to open the orifices and throughclear stasis. Rhinoceros Horn and Rehmannia Network-Quickening Beverage (*Xī Dì Qīng Luò Yǐn*) is a modified form of Rhinoceros Horn and Rehmannia Decoction (*Xī Jiǎo Dì Huáng Tāng*). In it:

§ Water buffalo horn (*shuǐ niú jiǎo*), moutan [root bark] (*dān pí*), raw rehmannia [root] (*shēng dì*), and raw red peony [root] (*shēng chì sháo*) (the ingredients of Rhinoceros Horn and Rehmannia

Decoction) are used as the principal ingredients, to cool and dissipate the blood.

§ Peach kernel (*táo rén*) and imperata [root] (*máo gēn*) are used to quicken blood and cool construction.

§ Forsythia [fruit] (*lián qiào*) and juncus (*dēng xīn*) are used to clear the heart and discharge heat.

§ Acorus [root] (*chāng pú*), dried bamboo sap (*zhú lì*), and ginger juice (*jiāng zhī*), are added as supplements, to flush phlegm and open the orifices.

When these medicinals are combined their overall effect is to clear and discharge the network vessel stasis and heat.

CHAPTER 12
AUTUMN DRYNESS

Autumn dryness is an externally contracted hot disease that occurs during autumn, and results from dry-heat disease pathogens. Initially, pathogens enter the lung defense and create symptoms such as dry throat, dry nose, coughing without much phlegm, and dry skin—characteristics of liquid *qì* dryness. Ordinarily, this disease is not too severe. Transmissions and changes are minimal and recovery is easy. Autumn dryness theory can be applied in pattern differentiation and treatment identification for biomedically defined conditions such as upper respiratory tract infections and acute bronchitis, particularly if they occur during autumn.

I. DISEASE CAUSES AND PATHOLOGY

The outbreak of this disease can be attributed to externally contracted dry-heat disease pathogens during autumn. The prevailing climate of autumn is sunny and dry. Therefore, during [early] autumn, when the weather tends to be sunny rather than rainy, overcast, and damp, externally contracted diseases usually manifest as warm dryness. During late autumn, on the other hand, when the whether tends to be somewhat cooler and the west wind is stronger, such diseases usually manifest as wind dryness (or as they are also called, cool dryness). This chapter, however, is limited to the discussion of warm dryness.

At the outbreak of this disease, pathogens are in the lung defense. Initially, therefore, its manifestations are similar to those of wind warmth, except that there are invariably accompanying patterns of dry liquid *qì*. This unique characteristic makes it easily distinguishable from the initial stages of other warm diseases.

Since dry *qì* easily consumes fluids, the initial manifestations of this disease include symptoms of dry liquid. Then, if rather than resolving, the lung defense pathogen transforms into heat and passes to the interior, the signs of dry liquid *qì* become even more prominent. Dry-heat in the lungs can easily dry the lungs and damage the *yīn*, but if it passes into the *yáng* brightness stomach and intestine, it commonly causes intestinal dryness constipation, or a vacuous *yīn* repletion bowel pattern. Normally, it never reaches the lower heater. Healthy resistance, or suitable treatments administered during its early stages, prevent it from doing so.

II. MAIN POINTS OF DIAGNOSIS

1. Initially, typical clinical characteristics include not only lung defense external patterns, but also dry mouth, nose, throat, and lips—symptoms of dried liquid *qì*.

2. There is a tendency for this pattern to occur during autumn when dry-heat is particularly exuberant.

3. The core of this disease is concentrated in the lungs. It is not very severe, and ordinarily its transmutations are minimal.

4. This disease must be differentiated from latent summerheat that occurs during autumn. In latent summerheat, although initially there are external patterns, the principal symptoms are of internal summerheat-damp. Also, the condition is more severe and the transformations are multitudinous.

III. PATTERN IDENTIFICATION AND TREATMENT DETERMINATION

Diseases caused by dry pathogens can easily damage the liquid, and as the *Classic of Internal Medicine* states in the *General Treatise on*

Essential Principles, "Dryness should be moistened." Hence when treating dryness the principal treatment policy is to enrich and moisten. Moreover, treatment books advise, "Treat the *qì* for upper dryness, increase the humor for middle dryness, and treat the blood for lower dryness."

These are the three main methods for treating the initial, middle, and final stages of autumn dryness. However it should not be forgotten that autumn dryness is an externally contracted dry *qì* disease. So initially, while external symptoms can be seen, although the principal treatment is to moisten the dryness, the secondary treatment must be to resolve the exterior according to pattern identification, so that the exterior pathogens can be outthrust. It is essential to use not only sweet moistening but also acrid cool medicinals.

It is also important to understand that dryness cannot be treated in the same way as fire. Generally, after a warm disease transforms into heat or fire, bitter cold heat-clearing and fire-draining methods are used. In dry patterns however, softening and moistening medicinals are usually indicated. Bitter drying medicinals are contraindicated. As our predecessors therefore said:

> *Fire can be treated by using bitter cold medicinals, dryness must be treated by using sweet cold medicinals; confined fire can be effused, victorious dryness must be moistened; fire can be curtailed directly, dryness must be moistened and nourished.*

Also, according to Wāng Sè Ān (汪瑟庵):

> *There are only a few methods for [managing] dry pattern, so their treatments are very simple. Initially, acrid cooling methods are used; then sweet cooling methods. These are similar to the normal treatments for warm heat. However, in the case of warm heat, when it passes into the middle burner, bitter cold supplements can be added, whereas in the case of dry patterns, softening moistening medicinals are normally indicated. Bitter drying medicinals are contraindicated.*

This is a very important guideline for clinical practice.

A. THE DISEASE PATTERN AND ITS TREATMENT IN LODGMENT OF PATHOGENS IN THE LUNG DEFENSE

Pattern

Fever, mild aversion to wind or cold, headache, scant sweating, coughing without much phlegm, dry throat, dry nose, thirst, white tongue moss, red tongue, and big rapid pulse on the right-hand side.

These symptoms occur at the initial stage of warm dryness, when pathogens raid the lung defense. Fever, mild aversion to wind and cold, headache, and scant sweating are evidence of dry-heat at the exterior. Coughing without much phlegm, dry throat, dry nose, and thirst are manifestations of dry-heat invading the lungs and damaging the lung liquid. White tongue moss, red tongue, and big rapid pulse are indications of dry-heat in the lung defense.

During their initial stages, this pattern and wind warmth are both similar because in both cases pathogens are in the lung defense. The main differences between them are that each of them is caused by a different pathogen and each occurs during a different season. Wind warmth results from a wind-heat pathogen and usually occurs during spring; this pattern results from a dry-heat pathogen and usually occurs during autumn. Clinically, therefore, this pattern manifests not only with basically the same external defense-exterior disease as wind warmth, but also with characteristic signs of dry-heat damaging the fluids. Consequently, they are not difficult to differentiate.

Treatment

Use acrid cool sweet moistening medicinals to lightly outthrust lung defense.

Prescriptions

Mulberry Leaf and Apricot Kernel Decoction
(*Sāng Xìng Tāng* 桑杏湯)

From the *Detailed Analysis of Warm Diseases* (*Wēn Bìng Tiáo Biàn* 溫病條辯)

mulberry leaf (*sāng yè*)	桑葉	3g
apricot kernel (*xìng rén*)	杏仁	5g
adenophora/glehnia [root] (*shā shēn*)	沙參	6g
Sichuan fritillaria [bulb] (*chuān bèi*)	川貝	3g
fermented soybean (*dòu chǐ*)	淡豆豉	3g
gardenia [fruit] peel (*zhī pí*)	梔皮	5g
pear peel (*lí pí*)	梨皮	3g

Boil in two cups of water until one cup is left and administer as soon as possible. In severe cases, give a second dose.

Since this pattern is caused by warm dryness raiding the lung defense, its treatment cannot be managed in the same way as either wind-cold or wind-heat. Neither acrid warming medicinals, nor unsupplemented acrid cooling medicinals are suitable. The only appropriate treatment is to cool the warmth while simultaneously moistening the dryness. This pattern must, in other words, be treated with acrid cool sweet moistening formulas. Mulberry Leaf and Apricot Kernel Decoction (*Sāng Xìng Tāng*) is a suitable prescription. In it:

- § Mulberry leaf (*sāng yè*), fermented soybean (*dòu chǐ*), and apricot kernel (*xìng rén*) diffuse the lungs and outthrust pathogens.
- § Fritillaria [bulb] (*bèi mǔ*) transforms phlegm.
- § Gardenia [fruit] peel (*zhī pí*) clears heat.
- § Adenophora/glehnia [root] (*shā shēn*) and pear peel (*lí pí*) nourish *yīn* and moisten dryness.

This enables pathogens to be eliminated without damage to the liquid. The overall effect of these ingredients is to course the exterior and moisten dryness.

B. Disease Patterns and Their Treatments in Lodgment of Pathogens in the *Qì* Aspect

1. Desiccation of the Clear Orifices

Pattern

Tinnitus, red eyes, swollen gums, and sore throat.

These are symptoms of upper burner *qì* aspect dry-heat harassing the clear orifices. The throat is the gateway of the lungs and stomach, and the gums correspond with the *yáng* brightness channel. Dry-heat follows the channel upward, so the throat is sore and the gums are swollen. The clear orifice is harassed so the ears are ringing and the eyes are red.

Treatment

Lightly clear, diffuse, and outthrust the upper burner *qì* aspect dry-heat.

Prescription

Forsythia and Mint Decoction (*Qiào Hé Tāng* 翹荷湯)
From the *Detailed Analysis of Warm Diseases* (*Wēn Bìng Tiáo Biàn* 溫病條辯).

mint (*bò hé*)	薄荷	5g
forsythia [fruit] (*lián qiào*)	連翹	10g
raw licorice [root] (*shēng gān cǎo*)	生甘草	5g
black gardenia [fruit] peel (*hēi zhī pī*)	黑梔皮	12g
platycodon [root] (*kǔ jié gěng*)	苦桔梗	6g
bean seed-coat (*lǜ dòu yī*)	綠豆衣	5g

Boil in two cups of water until one cup is left. Administer as soon as possible, and give twice daily or in severe cases three times a day.

Since this pattern occurs when dry-heat pathogens rise and dry, so that the clear orifices are inhibited and the disease is located above, and since the disease impetus is not very severe, the principal treatment is to lightly clear, diffuse, and outthrust the dry-heat from the upper burner. Forsythia and Mint Decoction (*Qiào Hé Tāng*) is a suitable mild acrid cool fire-clearing prescription, because in it:

§ Mint (*bò hé*), which has acrid cool properties, clears the head and eyes.

§ Forsythia [fruit] (*lián qiào*), black gardenia [fruit] peel (*hēi zhī pī*), and bean seed-coat (*lǜ dòu yī*) clear dry fire.

§ The combination of licorice [root] (*gān cǎo*) and platycodon [root] (*jié gěng*) disinhibits the throat and stops soreness.

2. DRY-HEAT DAMAGING THE LUNGS

Pattern

Fever, dry coughing without phlegm, *qì* counterflow dyspnea, dry throat, dry nose, fullness in the chest with rib-side pain, vexation and thirst, thick white dry tongue moss, and red tongue tip.

This pattern is characteristic of lung channel dry-heat transforming into fire and damaging the *yīn* humor. The lungs are scorched by heat and the lung *qì* loses its purifying function so fever, dry coughing without phlegm, and *qì* counterflow dyspnea occur. Heat congestion inhibits the *qì* dynamic so there is also fullness in the chest with rib-side pain. Although the *yīn* has been damaged by lung heat, the disease pathogen is still in the *qì* aspect, hence the tongue moss is thick, white, and dry, and the tongue tip is red.

Treatment

Clear the lung, moisten dryness, and nourish *yīn*.

Prescription

Dryness-Clearing Lung-Rescuing Decoction
(*Qīng Zào Jiù Fèi Tāng* 清燥救肺湯)

From the *Precepts for Physicians* (*Yī Mén Fǎ Lǜ* 醫門法律).

crude gypsum (*shēng shí gāo*)	生石膏	8g
frostbitten mulberry leaf (*dōng sāng yè*)	冬桑葉	10g
licorice [root] (*gān cǎo*)	甘草	3g
ginseng (*rén shēn*)	人參	2g
black sesame [seed] (*hú má rén*) (stir-bake and grind to powder)	胡麻仁	3g
aged ass hide glue (*chēn ē jiāo*)	真阿膠	3g
ophiopogon [tuber] (*mài mén dōng*) (remove core)	麥門冬	4g
apricot kernel (*xìng rén*) (remove skin and stir-bake)	杏仁	2g
loquat leaf (*pí pá yè*) (remove hairs and stir-bake in honey)	枇杷葉	3g

Boil in one cup of water until 60% is left. Give twice or three times daily.

Since this pattern occurs when dry-heat transforms into fire and damages the lung *yīn*, the principal treatment is to clear the lungs and moisten the dryness. Initially, the pathomechanism is centered in the *qì* rather than the blood aspect, so Dryness-Clearing Lung-Rescuing Decoction (*Qīng Zào Jiù Fèi Tāng*) is prescribed to clear and discharge lung heat, moisten dryness, and nourish lung *yīn*. In this formula:

§ Mulberry leaf (*sāng yè*), apricot kernel (*xìng rén*), and loquat leaf (*pí pá yè*) diffuse the lung and stop coughing.
§ Gypsum (*shí gāo*), licorice [root] (*gān cǎo*), and ophiopogon [tuber] (*mài dōng*) clear fire and engender liquid.
§ Ginseng (*rén shēn*) supplements and boosts the *qì* and *yīn*.
§ A combination of ass hide glue (*ē jiāo*) and hemp seed (*má rén*) enriches *yīn* and moistens dryness.

When these medicinals are combined, their overall effect is to clear the lung and moisten dryness. If the exterior muscles still contain pathogenic heat, it is important to consider adding light, diffusing supplements that are able to outthrust pathogens and discharge them from the exterior.

3. LUNG DRYNESS AND INTESTINAL HEAT WITH NETWORK VESSEL DAMAGE AND COUGHING OF BLOOD

Pattern

Initially there is itchy throat and dry coughing, then coughing of sticky phlegm which carries blood, pulling pains in the chest and rib-sides, scorching heat in the abdominal region, and diarrhea.

Initially, dry-heat damages the lungs causing itchy throat and dry coughing. Then dry-heat transforms into fire and scorches the lung network vessels, causing coughing of sticky phlegm which carries blood, and pulling pains in the chest and rib-sides. The lungs and the large intestines have an internal-external relationship. Lung heat shifts downward to the large intestines, so there is scorching heat in the abdominal region and diarrhea. Although watery, this diarrhea is accompanied by scorching pain at the anus or sometimes even in the abdomen, and like dysentery, it is difficult to pass. So it is different from vacuity cold diarrhea.

Treatment

Clear heat and stop bleeding, moisten the lungs and clear the intestines.

Prescription

Ass Hide Glue and Scutellaria Root Decoction
(*Ē Jiāo Huáng Qín Tāng* 阿膠黃芩湯)

From the *Popularized Treatise on Cold Damage* (*Tōng Sú Shāng Hán Lùn* 通俗傷寒論).

aged ass hide glue (*chén ē jiāo*)	陳阿膠	10g
[unripe] scutellaria [root] (*qīng zǐ qín*)	青子芩	10g
sweet apricot kernel (*tián xìng rén*)	甜杏仁	6g
raw mulberry root bark (*shēng sāng pí*)	生桑皮	6g
raw white peony [root] (*shēng bái sháo*)	生白芍	3g
raw licorice [root] (*shēng gān cǎo*)	生甘草	2g
fresh plantago (*xiān chē qián cǎo*)	鮮車前草	15g
sugar cane tips (*gān zhè shāo*)	甘蔗梢	15g

Boil the ingredients in water that has already been used to cook 30g of glutinous rice.

In this pattern lung dryness and intestinal heat cause diarrhea and coughing of blood, so treatment must be aimed at clearing heat and stopping bleeding, clearing the intestines and stopping diarrhea. In Ass Hide Glue and Scutellaria Root Decoction (*Ē Jiāo Huáng Qín Tāng*):

- § Sweet apricot kernel (*tián xìng rén*), raw mulberry root bark (*shēng sāng pí*), and sugar cane (*gān zhè*) moisten the lungs and engender liquid.
- § Ass hide glue (*ē jiāo*) nourishes blood and stops bleeding.
- § Raw white peony [root] (*shēng bái sháo*) and raw licorice [root] (*shēng gān cǎo*), which are sour and sweet, transform *yīn*, relax tension, and stop pain.
- § Scutellaria [root] (*huáng qín*) clears lung and large intestine heat.
- § Fresh plantago (*xiān chē qián cǎo*) abducts heat, downbears, and stops diarrhea.

4. DAMAGED LUNG AND STOMACH YĪN

Pattern

Fever that is not severe, non-stop dry coughing, dry mouth and tongue, and thirst.

This pattern occurs when scorching dry-heat damages the lung and stomach fluids. The lung liquid is damaged so there is non-stop coughing with scant phlegm. The stomach *yīn* is damaged so the mouth and tongue are both dry and there is thirst. The externally contracted pathogen is already cleaned, so the fever is not severe. Since the lung and stomach liquid has been damaged the tongue is usually red with scant moss.

Treatment

Enrich and moisten with sweet cold medicinals. Clear and nourish the lungs and stomach. Use Adenophora/Glehnia and Ophiopogon Decoction (*Shā Shēn Mài Mén Dōng Tāng* 沙參麥門冬湯), or if the liquid is severely damaged, Five Juices Beverage (*Wǔ Zhī Yīn* 五汁飲).

Prescriptions

Adenophora/Glehnia and Ophiopogon Decoction (*Shā Shēn Mài Mén Dōng Tāng* 沙參麥門冬湯) From the *Detailed Analysis of Warm Diseases* (*Wēn Bìng Tiáo Biàn* 溫病條辯).		
adenophora/glehnia [root] (*shā shēn*)	沙參	10g
Solomon's seal [root] (*yù zhú*)	玉竹	6g
raw licorice [root] (*shēng gān cǎo*)	生甘草	3g
frostbitten mulberry leaf (*dōng sāng yè*)	冬桑葉	5g
ophiopogon [tuber] (*mài dōng*)	麥冬	10g
raw lablab [bean] (*shēng biǎn dòu*)	生扁豆	5g
trichosanthes root (*huā fěn*)	花粉	5g

Boil all seven ingredients in five cups of water and simmer until two cups are left. Administer two doses per day, boiling the same packet of medicinals on both occasions.

Five Juices Beverage (*Wǔ Zhī Yǐn* 五汁飲) From the *Detailed Analysis of Warm Diseases* (*Wēn Bìng Tiáo Biàn* 溫病條辯).	
pear juice (*lí zhī*)	梨汁
water chestnut juice (*bí jì zhī*)	荸薺汁
fresh phragmites [root] juice (*xiān wěi gēn zhī*)	鮮葦根汁
fresh ophiopogon [tuber] juice (*mài dōng zhī*)	麥冬汁
lotus root juice (*ǒu zhī*)	藕汁

Give whenever necessary, as much as necessary, warm or cold.

This is a pattern in which dry-heat is not very severe. Its principal characteristic is damaged liquid, so treatment must focus on enriching and nourishing the lung and stomach fluids.

In Adenophora/Glehnia and Ophiopogon Decoction (*Shā Shēn Mài Mén Dōng Tāng*):

§ Adenophora/glehnia [root] (*shā shēn*), ophiopogon [tuber] (*mài dōng*), trichosanthes root (*tiān huā fěn*), and Solomon's seal [root] (*yù zhú*) enrich and nourish lung and stomach *yīn*.

§ Lablab [bean] (*biǎn dòu*) and licorice [root] (*gān cǎo*) harmonize and nourish stomach *qì*.

§ Mulberry leaf (*sāng yè*) clears and discharges pathogenic heat.

In cases where damaged liquid is accompanied by more severe thirst, prescribe Five Juices Beverage (*Wǔ Zhī Yǐn*) instead. This formula engenders liquid and nourishes humor, and moistens dryness and stops thirst.

5. LUNG DRYNESS AND INTESTINAL BLOCK

Pattern

Muted coughing of copious phlegm, chest and abdomen fullness and distention, and constipation.

In this pattern, although the exterior pathogens have already resolved, the lungs are affected with dry damage—so the *qì* dynamic loses uninhibited diffusion, and consequently there is muted coughing. When the lungs are damaged by dry-heat they lose their distributing function. Instead of circulating, fluids gather, so coughing produces copious phlegm. The lungs are unable to disseminate liquid, so the large intestines lose moisture, the dregs gather internally, and there is constipation with abdominal distention. These symptoms are indicative of both lung and large intestine diseases.

Treatment

Depurate the lungs and transform phlegm. Moisten the intestines and throughclear stools.

Prescription

Five-Kernel Tangerine Peel Decoction (*Wǔ Rén Jú Pí Tāng* 五仁桔皮湯)

From the *Popularized Treatise on Cold Damage* (*Tōng Sú Shāng Hán Lùn* 通俗傷寒論).

sweet apricot kernel (*tián xìng rén*) (crush)	甜杏仁	10g
pine nut (*sōng zǐ rén*)	松子仁	10g
bush cherry kernel (*yù lǐ rén*) (crush)	鬱李仁	13g
unhusked peach kernel (*yuán táo rén*) (crush)	原桃仁	6g
biota seed (*bǎi zǐ rēn*)	柏子仁	6g
tangerine peel (*jú pí*) (stir-bake with honey)	桔皮	5g

In this pattern, constipation results because the lungs are dry, the intestines are blocked, and the fluids are insufficient. It is therefore different from a *yáng* brightness repletion dryness stagnant bind pattern. Bitter cold downward-attacking prescriptions such as the *Qì*-Infusing Decoctions (*Chéng Qì Tāng*) are unsuitable, so Five-Kernel Tangerine Peel Decoction (*Wǔ Rén Jú Pí Tāng*), which depurates the lungs and transforms phlegm, moistens the intestines and throughclears stools, is used instead. In this formula:

§ Pine nut (*sōng zǐ rén*), bush cherry kernel (*yù lǐ rén*), peach kernel (*táo rén*), and biota seed (*bǎi zǐ rēn*), which are all rich in oils, moisten dryness and lubricate the intestines.

- § Sweet apricot kernel (*tián xìng rén*) moistens the lungs and transforms phlegm, lubricates the intestines and throughclears the stools.
- § Tangerine peel (*jú pí*) moves *qì* and eliminates distention.

Stir-baking tangerine peel in honey enriches its moisture and prevents it from drying. The overall effect of these six medicinals is to open the lungs and moisten the dryness. Since the lungs and the large intestines have an internal-external relationship, as soon as the lung *qì* is once more able to downbear, the stools are easily throughcleared.

6. BOWEL REPLETION AND YĪN DAMAGE

Pattern

Constipation, abdominal distention, fever, sometimes clouded spirit with delirious speech, and dry black tongue moss.

Yáng brightness heat bind damages liquid and causes *qì* to stagnate, so the stools fail to throughclear and the abdomen grows distended and full. Stomach heat harasses and confuses the spirit light so fever results, and sometimes unclear spirit knowledge with delirious speech. Heat bind at the interior covers and scorches the fluids so the tongue moss appears dry and black.

Although this and the immediately preceding pattern are both characterized by constipation, each has a different pathomechanism. In lung dryness and intestinal block, the lungs are unable to disseminate liquid so the intestines dry and there is constipation. But the spirit is not clouded, the speech is not delirious, and the tongue moss is not dry and black—there are no symptoms of internal exuberant pathogenic heat. In this pattern, dry-heat binds and stagnates, so the bowels become replete and the *yīn* is damaged. But there is no coughing of copious phlegm—lung patterns can not be seen. These are the important points of differentiation.

Treatment

Nourish *yīn* and downward-throughclear.

Prescriptions

Stomach-Regulating Qì-Infusing Decoction
(*Tiáo Wèi Chéng Qì Tāng* 調胃承氣湯)
Supplemented with fresh flowery knotweed [root] (*xiān shǒu wū* 鮮首烏), fresh raw rehmannia [root] (*xiān shēng dì* 鮮生地), and fresh dendrobium [stem] (*xiān shí hú* 鮮石斛).

From the *Treatise on Cold Damage* (*Shāng Hán Lùn* 傷寒論).

honey-fried licorice [root] (*zhì gān cǎo*)	炙甘草	60g
mirabilite (*máng xiāo*)	芒硝	240g
rhubarb (*dà huáng*) (wash with alcohol)	大黃	120g
fresh flowery knotweed [root] (*xiān shǒu wū*)	鮮首烏	150g
fresh raw rehmannia [root] (*xiān shēng dì*)	鮮生地	200g
fresh dendrobium [stem] (*xiān shí hú*)	鮮石斛	100g

In this pattern, since dry-heat binds internally, the treatment should aim to attack below; and since the fluids suffer damage, it ought also to aim at enriching *yīn*. Therefore Stomach-Regulating Qì-Infusing Decoction (*Tiáo Wèi Chéng Qì Tāng*) is used to attack and expel pathogenic heat, while fresh flowery knotweed [root] (*xiān shǒu wū*), fresh raw rehmannia [root] (*xiān shēng dì*), and fresh dendrobium [stem] (*xiān shí wú*) are added to enrich and nourish the fluids. Downward-throughclearing preserves *yīn*, and enriching *yīn* helps downward-throughclearing. So by using these methods together, bowel repletion is eliminated and *yīn* liquid is restored.

CHAPTER 13
WARM TOXICITY

Warm toxicity is contracted from warm heat toxin pathogens and is a type of warm heat seasonal toxin disease. Usually it is characterized by local redness, swelling, and pain, or sometimes even open ulcerations, and initially it is accompanied by external patterns.

Records show that although warm toxicity has been used as a term from very ancient times, it has only been used with any sense of specificity from the Qīng Dynasty. Wú Jú Tōng declared:

> *Warm toxicity is marked by sore swollen throat, swelling anterior and posterior to the ear, cheek swelling, and red complexion, or throat not sore but [with] external swelling, and in severe cases deafness.*

This describes the clinical manifestations of warm toxicity. Léi Shào Yì (雷少逸) contributed further by adding, "Warm toxicity can also cause macular eruptions, papular eruptions, jowl effusions, and throat swellings that must be understood." Even now, warm toxicity is generally not used as a term for a specific disease, but as a general term for a wide range of diseases with similar characteristics—diseases such as massive head scourge[1], putrefying throat eruptions[2], throat-entwining wind,[3] and swollen cheeks[4]. Warm toxicity theory can be applied in pattern differentiation and treatment identification

[1] "Massive head scourge" is a traditional name for erysipelas.
[2] "Putrefying throat eruptions" is a traditional name for scarlet fever.
[3] "Throat-entwining wind" is a traditional name for diphtheria.
[4] "Swollen cheeks" is a traditional name for epidemic parotitis (i.e., mumps).

of biomedically defined conditions such as erysipelas, scarlet fever, diphtheria, and epidemic parotitis. Since certain of these diseases, like throat-entwining wind and swollen cheeks, are primarily pediatric diseases, this chapter deals only with massive head scourge and putrefying throat eruptions.

MASSIVE HEAD SCOURGE

The name of this disease is derived from the fact that after pathogens are contracted, the head and face become red and swollen. In addition, since at its onset there are usually exterior symptoms such as fever and aversion to cold, which are symptoms similar to those of cold damage, it is also called "massive head cold damage." Since it is externally contracted it is also called "wind warmth seasonal toxin." And when head and face swelling develop very quickly, like moving wind, it is also called "massive head wind"or "wind warmth seasonal toxicity."

I. DISEASE CAUSES AND PATHOLOGY

The main cause of this disease is an externally contracted warm heat toxin pathogen. Outbreaks usually occur during spring, when wind warmth grows abnormally intense, or during winter when the whether which is normally cold turns unseasonably hot, and it easily enters the body when pathogens are contracted during insufficiency of right *qì*. The main pathomechanical transformations are caused by pathogens invading the defense *qì*, and heat toxins flooding the lungs and stomach.

Initially the toxin pathogens are mild, and the defense aspect is invaded, so during the onset an exterior defense disease can be seen. During the following stage, heat toxins slowly intensify, passing from the defense aspect to the *qì* aspect, searing and scorching the lungs and stomach so that symptoms of exuberant lung and stomach heat appear. Pathogen toxins attack the head and face. Thrusting at and binding to the throat, they cause local redness, swelling, soreness, and, in severe cases, open ulcerations.

II. MAIN POINTS OF DIAGNOSIS

1. Whenever symptoms of redness, swelling, and soreness at the head and face develop rapidly during winter or spring, this disease must be suspected.

2. In massive head scourge there is very little variation in the systemic patterns. The pathogens seldom if ever fall into the construction and blood aspects.

3. This disease must be differentiated from swollen cheeks (i.e., mumps). In this disease the principal symptom is redness and swelling of the head and face; in mumps there is swelling at one or both parotid glands—below and in front of the ears. Also, when heat toxins penetrate below, there can be orchitis.

III. PATTERN IDENTIFICATION AND TREATMENT DETERMINATION

Pattern

Initially there is fever, abhorrence of cold, redness and swelling at the head and face, and sore throat. Subsequently there is slowly diminishing aversion to cold with slowly increasing fever, thirst with desire to drink, vexation and agitation, scorching-hot swollen head and face, increased throat soreness, red tongue with yellow moss, and rapid replete pulse.

Warm toxin pathogens accompany external contraction and are normally confined at the exterior muscles. The defense *qì* loses harmony, so initially external symptoms such as aversion to cold and fever can be seen. All *yáng* channels connect at the head, so when heat toxins attack above the head and face become red and swollen or the throat becomes sore. When warm toxins transform into fire, pathogenic heat gradually enters deeper, flooding the lungs and stomach. The pattern, which was previously mild, becomes severe. Rather than remaining resident in the exterior defense, pathogenic heat passes to the *qì* aspect. Consequently, aversion to cold slowly diminishes, and fever slowly increases. As *qì* aspect heat intensifies it begins to damage the fluids. Thus, as the heat dynamic invigorates, thirst, vexation, and agitation develop. Heat toxins flood the head and face, so soreness and swelling of the throat increases. Red tongue, yellow tongue moss, and rapid replete pulse are characteristic of exuberant internal heat.

Treatment

Course wind and clear heat. Resolve toxins and disperse swelling. Internally, give Universal Salvation Toxin-Dispersing Beverage (*Pŭ Jì Xiāo Dú Yĭn*); externally, apply Three Yellows and Two Fragrances Powder (*Sān Huáng Èr Xiāng Săn*).

Prescriptions

Universal Salvation Toxin-Dispersing Beverage (*Pŭ Jì Xiāo Dú Yĭn* 普濟消毒飲)

From *Dōng Yuán's Ten Books* (*Dōng Yuán Shí Shū* 東垣十書).

scutellaria [root] (*huáng qín*)	黄芩	6g
coptis [root] (*huáng lián*)	黄連	2g
scrophularia [root] (*xuán shēn*)	玄参	10g
forsythia [fruit] (*lián qiào*)	連翹	10g
isatis root (*băn lán gēn*)	板籃根	10g
puffball (*mă bó*)	馬勃	5g
arctium [seed] (*niú bàng zĭ*)	牛蒡子	10g
mint (*bò hé*)	薄荷	3g
silkworm (*jiāng cán*)	僵蠶	6g
platycodon [root] (*kŭ jié gĕng*)	苦桔梗	3g
cimicifuga [root] (*shēng má*)	升麻	2g
bupleurum [root] (*chái hú*)	柴胡	3g
tangerine peel (*chén pí*)	陳皮	5g
raw licorice [root] (*shēng gān căo*)	生甘草	3g

Three Yellows and Two Fragrances Powder (*Sān Huáng Èr Xiāng Săn* 三黄二香散)

From the *Detailed Analysis of Warm Diseases* (*Wēn Bìng Tiáo Biàn* 溫病條辯).

coptis [root] (*huáng lián*)	黄連	30g
phellodendron [bark] (*huáng băi*)	黄柏	30g
raw rhubarb (*shēng dà huáng*)	生大黄	30g
frankincense (*rŭ xiāng*)	乳香	15g
myrrh (*mò yào*)	沒藥	15g

Grind all ingredients into a powder, mix them with tea, wait until they dry, and then mix in sesame oil.

In Universal Salvation Toxin-Dispersing Beverage (*Pŭ Jì Xiāo Dú Yĭn*):

§ Mint (*bò hé*), arctium [seed] (*niú bàng zĭ*), silkworm (*jiāng cán*), and bupleurum [root] (*chái hú*), all of which are acrid and cool, diffusing and outthrusting, resolve external pathogenic heat from the defense aspect.

§ Scutellaria [root] (*huáng qín*) and coptis [root] (*huáng lián*), both of which are bitter and cold, clear *qì* aspect fire heat.

§ Cimicifuga [root] (*shēng má*), forsythia [fruit] (*lián qiào*), isatis root (*bǎn lán gēn*), puffball (*mǎ bó*), licorice [root] (*gān cǎo*), and platycodon [root] (*jié gěng*), all of which are heat-clearing and pharynx disinhibiting, resolve toxins and disperse swelling.

§ Scrophularia [root] (*xuán shēn*), which is salty and cold, engenders liquid and restrains pathogenic fire.

When these medicinals are combined, their overall effect is to course, outthrust, clear, and resolve—to scatter and disperse both internally and externally. When used clinically, this prescription is modified to suit the condition. Initially, when pathogens tend to fix in the defense exterior, add schizonepeta (*jīng jiè*) and ledebouriella [root] (*fáng fēng*), which are acrid and dissipating, to strengthen the exterior-outthrusting pathogen-coursing functions. Later, when the internal heat is already exuberant and there is bowel repletion constipation, add medicinals like raw rhubarb (*shēng dà huáng*), which throughclears the bowel and discharges heat, to induce downward discharge of heat toxins.

Three Yellows and Two Fragrances Powder (*Sān Huáng Èr Xiāng Sǎn*) is an externally applied formula for treating local redness, swelling, heat, and pain (i.e., soreness). It contains coptis [root] (*huáng lián*), phellodendron [bark] (*huáng bǎi*), raw rhubarb (*dà huáng*), frankincense (*rǔ xiāng*), and myrrh (*mò yào*). All of the "three yellow" medicinals—coptis [root] (*huáng lián*), phellodendron [bark] (*huáng bǎi*), and raw rhubarb (*dà huáng*)—are bitter, cold, and heat-clearing, so all three downbear fire and resolve toxins. Frankincense (*rǔ xiāng*) and myrrh (*mò yào*) are acrid, bitter, and slightly warming. They quicken blood and scatter stasis, disperse swelling and settle pain. When these medicinals are combined, their overall effect is to clear fire, resolve toxins, disperse swelling, and stop pain.

PUTREFYING THROAT ERUPTIONS

Putrefying throat eruptions is [a condition] associated with contraction of warm heat toxin pathogens and is characterized by swelling and soreness of the throat with scarlet skin eruptions. Since it usually occurs during winter and spring, when the weather grows suddenly warmer, it is sometimes called "seasonal throat eruptions." Being extremely contagious, it is also known as "epidemic throat eruptions." These names reflect its clinical characteristics, its seasonal nature, and the fact that it is influenced by the prevailing weather conditions. In biomedicine it is called scarlet fever.

I. DISEASE CAUSES AND PATHOLOGY

This disease is caused mainly by externally contracted warm toxin pathogens. Disease pathogens usually enter via the mouth and nose, and are more readily contracted by people with pre-existing *yīn* vacuity. The main pathomechanism is that warm toxins, which invade the exterior, are contracted by the lungs and stomach. The throat is the gateway to the lungs and stomach. Consequently, when heat toxins rise and drench, in mild cases there will be unbearably sore swollen throat; in severe cases there will be erosions with oozing of blood.

The lungs govern the skin and hair; the stomach governs the muscles. Therefore, when heat toxins surface externally to the muscles and skin from the lungs and stomach, the whole body is covered in scarlet eruptions that are as numerous as the stars in the sky, as smooth as pieces of satin. Initially, this disease usually presents with defense aspect external symptoms. Then, as the pathogen enters from the exterior to the interior, exuberant *qì* aspect heat is usually seen; and as heat toxins drive internally, towards the construction-blood, severe symptoms at both the *qì* and construction (blood) aspects can appear. If there are myriad ulcers at the isthmus of fauces, the airways are obstructed and blocked, the eruptions are purple red, the spirit is clouded, and the tongue is crimson, then the pattern is very severe. During the final stage the *yīn* liquid is detrimented, and residual pathogens linger, so usually there are symptoms of residual toxins damaging *yīn*.

II. MAIN POINTS OF DIAGNOSIS

1. The keys to diagnosing this disease are knowing that it normally occurs during winter and spring, that there is always a history of contact with other infected people, and that there are always symptoms of acute fever, sore swollen eroded throat, myriad skin eruptions, and crimson tongue.

2. During the course of the disease, heat toxins usually enter deeply and strong symptoms such as high fever, myriad purple black eruptions, and extremely sore eroded throat occur. These are severe symptoms of heat toxins scorching the *qì* and blood. If sore throat and erosion are not very severe, but are accompanied by myriad dull purple eruptions, high fever, clouded spirit, limb reversal (manifesting primarily as cold limbs), and sunken fine pulse, internal block and external desertion is indicated. This is a critical condition.

3. This disease, diphtheria, and measles all generally occur during the same seasons (i.e., winter and spring). It is therefore important they be differentiated. In "white throat" (i.e., diphtheria), there are no papules and the sore swollen throat is easily recognized because it is characteristically covered by a white membrane-like coating. In measles, papules appear as tiny points or join together into patches and protrude above the level of the skin. There are also rashes in the throat that can be blood-engorged and painful, but there is never erosion. Checking for these characteristics makes differentiation easy.

III. PATTERN IDENTIFICATION AND TREATMENT DETERMINATION

The main treatment principle for this disease must be to clear and discharge pathogen toxins. In clinical practice, however, different methods are used for different stages, different locations (whether shallow or deep), and different conditions (whether mild or severe). Initially, while the pathogen is still in the defense exterior and the condition is not very severe, acrid cool diffusing-discharging methods must be used to outthrust the exterior pathogens. Later, after disease pathogens pass to the interior, and increased heat transforms into fire, fire-clearing toxin-resolving methods must be used. When a pathogen is prominently in the *qì* aspect, the main aim of treatment must be to clear *qì*. When it enters the construction-blood, the main aim must be to clear construction and cool blood. When it is strong at both the *qì* and construction-blood aspects, the aim must be to clear *qì* while simultaneously cooling construction-blood. During the final stage, when the construction *yīn* has been damaged, the main aim must be to clear construction and nourish *yīn*.

A. TOXINS INVADING THE LUNG DEFENSE

Pattern

Aversion to cold and fever, headache and body pain, slight thirst, sore red swollen throat or throat erosion, eruptions, red tongue, thin white non-moist tongue moss, and floating rapid pulse.

This pattern can be seen during the initial stage of putrefying throat eruptions. The principal pathomechanism is loss of lung defense function, so symptoms of pathogenic heat in the external defense aspect, such as fever and aversion to cold, headache and body pains, thirst, thin white dry tongue moss, and floating rapid pulse appear. The throat is the gateway of the lungs and stomach. Therefore, when lung and stomach heat toxins drench above, the throat becomes sore, red, swollen, and eroded. The reason that eruptions can be seen is that pathogen toxins are attempting to surface through to the muscles and skin. Since this pattern is characterized by these local symptoms and by symptoms of toxins attacking the lung defense, it is easily distinguishable from other warm diseases.

Treatment

Course the exterior and diffuse the lungs. Discharge heat and resolve toxins. Internally, give Throat-Clearing Decoction (*Qīng Yān Tāng*); externally, apply Jade Key (*Yù Yào Shí*).

Prescriptions

Throat-Clearing Decoction (*Qīng Yān Tāng* 清咽湯)

From *Treatise on Epidemic Throat Diseases with Simple Explanations* (*Yì Hóu Qiǎn Lùn* 疫喉淺論)

schizonepeta (*jīng jiè*)	荆芥	5g
ledebouriella [root] (*fáng fēng*)	防風	5g
platycodon [root] (*jié gěng*)	桔梗	5g
apricot kernel (*xìng rén*)	杏仁	10g

licorice [root] (*gān cǎo*)	甘草	3g
bitter orange (*zhǐ qiào*)	枳殼	3g
fresh duckweed (*xiān fú píng*)	鮮浮萍	3g
peucedanum [root] (*qián hú*)	前胡	5g
arctium [seed] (*niú bàng zǐ*)	牛蒡子	3g
silkworm (*bái jiāng cán*)	白僵蠶	6g
Chinese olive (*gǎn lǎn*)	橄欖	3 seeds
mint (*bò hé*)	薄荷	3g

Jade Key (*Yù Yào Shí* 玉鑰匙)

From the *Pattern Treatment Criterion* (*Zhèng Zhì Zhǔn Shéng* 證治準繩)

niter (*yàn xiāo*)	焰硝	45g
borax (*péng shā*)	硼砂	15g
borneol (*nǎo zǐ*)	腦子	10g
silkworm (*bái jiāng cán*)	白僵蠶	8g

Grind all the ingredients into a fine powder and blow it onto the throat.

In Throat-Clearing Decoction (*Qīng Yān Tāng*):

- § Schizonepeta (*jīng jiè*), ledebouriella [root] (*fáng fēng*), mint (*bò hé*), and fresh duckweed (*xiān fú píng*), all of which are acrid and resolving, outthrusting and outpushing exterior pathogens.
- § Apricot kernel (*xìng rén*), bitter orange (*zhǐ qiào*), and platycodon [root] (*jié gěng*), all of which diffuse and open lung *qì*, assist in outpushing pathogens to the exterior.
- § Arctium [seed] (*niú bàng zǐ*), silkworm (*jiāng cán*), Chinese olive (*gǎn lǎn*), and raw licorice [root] (*shēng gān cǎo*) all clear heat, resolve toxins, and disinhibit the throat.

The overall effect of this combination is to diffuse the exterior and resolve toxins—it resolves pathogen toxins at the exterior. As the medical expert Dīng Gān Rén (丁甘仁) said, "In putrefying throat eruptions the most important criteria is to enable convenient sweating." And as Chén Gēng Dào (陳耕道) advised:

> *For pathogens at the exterior, course and outpush. . . . Fire is not scorching internally so eruptions do not reflect severe heat, spirits are clear, and throats are not eroded. As a general rule, first outthrust and later clear.*

Both these passages note that during the initial stage of this disease it is very important to treat by resolving the exterior and outthrusting the pathogens.

Jade Key *(Yù Yào Shí)* is a commonly used external treatment for throat diseases. Its ingredients clear heat and disinhibit the throat, disperse swelling and stabilize pain. It is therefore effective whenever there is red swollen sore throat.

B. TOXINS OBSTRUCTING THE *QÌ* ASPECT

Pattern

Vigorous fever, vexation and agitation, thirst with desire to drink, red swollen eroded throat, manifesting of scattered eruptions, red tongue with dry yellow moss, and surging rapid pulse.

This pattern usually develops when the immediately preceding pattern progresses from shallow to deep, from the defense to the *qì*, and heat toxins gradually grow exuberant. The pathomechanism inclines to heat congesting and obstructing the *qì* aspect, so clinical manifestations of interior heat such as vigorous fever, vexation and thirst, and surging pulse can be seen. Since intensely exuberant heat toxins drench above, fuming and scorching the lung and stomach throughconnecting path, the throat is sore, swollen, and eroded. Since they surface to the muscle and skin through the blood network vessels, eruptions occur.

Treatment

Clear *qì* and resolve toxins.

Prescriptions

Yú's Heart-Clearing Diaphragm-Cooling Powder
(*Yú Shì Qīng Xīn Liáng Gé Săn* 余氏清心涼膈散)
From *Warm Heat Latitudes and Longitudes* (*Wēn Rè Jīng Wěi* 温热经纬).

forsythia [fruit] (*lián qiào*)	連翹	10g
scutellaria [root] (*huáng qín*)	黄芩	10g
gardenia [fruit] (*shān zhī*)	山梔	10g
mint (*bò hé*)	薄荷	3g
gypsum (*shí gāo*)	石膏	20g
platycodon [root] (*kŭ jié gěng*)	苦桔梗	3g
licorice [root] (*gān căo*)	甘草	3g

Tin-Like Powder (*Xí Lèi Săn* 錫類散)		
From the *Golden Chamber Wings* (*Jīn Kuì Yì* 金匱翼).		
ivory flakes (*xiàng yá xiè*) (bake over a slow fire)	象牙屑	1.5g
pearl (*zhēn zhū*) (process)	珍珠	1.5g
indigo (*qīng dài*) (elutriate)	青黛	1.5g
borneol (*bīng piàn*)	冰片	0.5g
wall spider (*bì qián*) (from mud-brick walls)	壁錢	20
bovine bezoar (*niú huáng*)	牛黄	0.7g
stone-baked nail clippings (*bèi zhĭ jiă*)	焙指甲	0.7g

Grind all the ingredients into a fine powder and store them in a small airtight bottle. At each application, blow small quantities of this powder onto the throat.

Yú's Heart-Clearing Diaphragm-Cooling Powder (*Yú Shì Qīng Xīn Liáng Gé Săn*) cools the diaphragm and discharges heat. In it:

- § Forsythia [fruit] (*lián qiào*), scutellaria [root] (*huáng qín*), and gardenia [fruit] (*shān zhī*) clear heat and cool the diaphragm.
- § Gypsum (*shí gāo*) and mint (*bò hé*), being acrid and cooling, outthrust heat.
- § Licorice [root] (*gān căo*) and platycodon [root] (*jié gĕng*) clear and disinhibit the throat.

Tin-Like Powder (*Xí Lèi Săn*) is particularly good at clearing heat and resolving toxins, but can also eliminate the putrid and engender soft tissue. It is therefore an ideal formula for throat putrefying.

C. TOXINS FLARING IN THE *QÌ* AND CONSTRUCTION [BLOOD] ASPECTS

Pattern

High fever, vexation and agitation, thirst, red swollen eroded throat that in severe cases obstructs the airways, mute voice and tachypnea, myriad concentrated purple-red joined-together skin eruptions, dry crimson tongue with numerous thorns, and fine rapid pulse.

By this stage putrefying throat eruptions are extremely severe. Warm toxin pathogens transform into dryness and fire, so redness, swelling, and throat erosion can be seen. Heat flares in the *qì* aspect, so high fever, vexation, and thirst are manifest. Heat fumes and scorches the construction [blood] aspect, so myriad concentrated, dark-black joined-together skin eruptions occur. And heat toxins damage the construction so the tongue has a dry, crimson-red appearance with numerous thorns. This pattern is the most severe manifestation of toxins congesting the *qì* aspect—the disease is deeper [than before] and the condition is extremely dangerous.

Treatment

Clear both the *qì* and construction.Resolve the toxins and rescue the *yīn*.

Prescription

Construction-Cooling Qì-Clearing Decoction
(*Liáng Yíng Qīng Qì Tāng* 凉营清气汤)
From *Dīng Gān Rén's Case Histories* (*Dīng Gān Rén Yī Àn* 丁甘仁醫案)

rhinoceros horn tip (*xī jiǎo jiān*) (ground into powder)	犀角尖	2g
fresh dendrobium [stem] (*xiān shí hú*)	鮮石斛	26g
black gardenia (*hēi zhī*)	黑梔	5g
moutan [root bark] (*dān pí*)	丹皮	5g
fresh raw rehmannia [root] (*xiān shēng dì*)	鮮生地	26g
mint leaf (*bò hé yè*)	薄荷葉	3g
Sichuan coptis [root] (*chuān lián*)	川連	3g
red peony [root] (*chì sháo*)	赤芍	5g
scrophularia [root] (*xuán shēn*)	玄參	10g
crude gypsum (*shēng shí gāo*)	生石膏	25g
raw licorice [root] (*shēng gān cǎo*)	生甘草	3g
fresh bamboo leaf (*xiān zhú yè*)	鮮竹葉	30pc
forsythia [fruit] shell (*lián qiào qiào*)	連翹殼	10g
phragmites [root] (*lú gēn*)	蘆根	30g
imperata [root] (*máo gēn*)	茅根	30g
purified feces (*jīn zhī*) (mix in after decoction is ready)	金汁	30g

These days, use 6g of water buffalo horn (*shuǐ niú jiǎo*) instead of 2g of rhinoceros horn tip (*xī jiǎo jiān*), and omit purified feces (*jīn zhī*).

This formula is made by combining Jade Lady Brew (*Yù Nǚ Jiān*), Diaphragm-Cooling Powder (*Liáng Gé Sǎn*), and Construction-Clearing Decoction (*Qīng Yíng Tāng*). In it:

§ Water buffalo horn (*shuǐ niú jiǎo*), fresh raw rehmannia [root] (*xiān shēng dì*), moutan [root bark] (*dān pí*), and red peony

[root] (*chì sháo*) resolve toxins by clearing construction and cooling blood.

§ Gardenia [fruit] (*zhī zǐ*), mint (*bò hé*), forsythia [fruit] (*lián qiào*), gypsum (*shí gāo*), coptis [root] (*huáng lián*), and licorice [root] (*gān cǎo*) clear *qì*, discharge heat, and resolve toxins.

§ Dendrobium [stem] (*shí hú*), bamboo leaf (*zhú yè*), scrophularia [root] (*xuán shēn*), phragmites [root] (*lú gēn*), and imperata [root] (*bái máo gēn*), all of which are sweet and cold, rescue *yīn* by engendering liquid and nourishing humor.

The overall function of this combination is to clear heat and resolve toxins, cool construction and engender liquid.

In more severe conditions there will be symptoms of internal block and external desertion, symptoms such as clouded spirit, delirious speech, dyspnea, coughing, verging on desertion, limb reversal (manifesting primarily as cold limbs), and hidden pulse. In these cases use medicinals that rescue counterflow and stem desertion, such as ginseng (*rén shēn*), aconite [accessory tuber] (*fù zǐ*), dragon bone (*lóng gǔ*), and oyster shell (*mǔ lì*), in combination with prescriptions that clear the heart and open the orifice, such as Peaceful Palace Bovine Bezoar Pill (*Ān Gōng Niú Huáng Wán*). Do not use Construction-Cooling *Qì*-Clearing Decoction (*Liáng Yíng Qīng Qì Tāng*) until after the condition improves.

D. REMNANT TOXINS INJURING YĪN

Pattern

Sore swollen throat with less severe erosions, skin eruptions scattering and abating, diminished vigorous fever with only low fever in the afternoon still occurring, dry mouth, heat in the centers of the palms and soles, fine rapid pulse, and dry red tongue.

This pattern is commonly seen during the recovery stage of putrefying throat eruptions—when the pathogen toxins have been reduced but their remnants are still lingering. The vigorous fever has already abated, but the *yīn* liquid has not yet restored, so there are *yīn* vacuity internal heat symptoms such as afternoon fevers, dry mouth, heat in the centers of the palms and soles, fine rapid pulse, and dry tongue. The less severe throat erosions indicate that remnant toxins are no longer causing vigorous disease. It is therefore important not only to monitor the disease progress, but also to differentiate its primary and secondary clinical manifestations. In this condition, the pathomechanism tends towards vacuity and damage to the *yīn* liquid. Since the *yīn* humor has not yet restored and the heat has not yet completely abated and cleared, the symptoms have not yet dispersed and eliminated.

Treatment

Nourish yīn and engender liquid. Clear and depurate remnant toxins.

Prescription

Throat-Clearing Construction-Nourishing Decoction
(*Qīng Yān Yǎng Yíng Tāng* 清咽養營湯)
From the *Treatise on Epidemic Throat Diseases* (*Yì Hóu Qiǎn Lùn* 疫喉淺論)

American ginseng (*xī yáng shēn*)	西洋參	10g
thick raw rehmannia [root] (*dà shēng dì*)	大生地	10g
root poria (*fú shén*)	茯神	10g
ophiopogon [tuber] (*mài dōng*)	麥冬	10g
white peony [root] (*bái sháo*)	白芍	5g
trichosanthes root (*huā fěn*)	花粉	12g
asparagus [tuber] (*tiān dōng*)	天冬	5g
scrophularia [root] (*xuán shēn*)	玄參	12g
anemarrhena [root] (*zhī mǔ*)	知母	10g
honey-fried licorice [root] (*zhì gān cǎo*)	炙甘草	3g

In this prescription:

§ American ginseng (*xī yáng shēn*) (or adenophora/glehnia [root] (*shā shēn*), which is a suitable substitute), ophiopogon [tuber] (*mài dōng*), and raw rehmannia [root] (*shēng dì*) are used as emperor medicinals to nourish *yīn* and increase humor.

§ Asparagus [tuber] (*tiān dōng*), scrophularia [root] (*xuán shēn*), white peony [root] (*bái sháo*) and licorice [root] (*gān cǎo*) which are sour, sweet, and *yīn*-transforming are used as ministers to strengthen the functions of the emperor medicinals by nourishing humor and engendering liquid.

§ Anemarrhena [root] (*zhī mǔ*) and trichosanthes root (*huā fěn*) are used to clear and discharge the remnant heat.

§ Root poria (*fú shén*) is used to nourish the heart and quiet the spirit.

ENGLISH, CHINESE, AND *PĪNYĪN* GLOSSARY OF UNCOMMON CHINESE MEDICAL TERMS

Abhorrence of cold: *zēng hán* 憎寒. This term has the same meaning as aversion to cold.

Confined: *yù* 郁. *Yù* means "confined" and also "gloomy." Of these meanings we consider "confined" to be the most pertinent and so have used it as our translation. "Confined" is not a word used to describe any other specific medical phenomena, so it does not have the potential to cause unnecessary confusion.

Core of pathogenic change: *bìng biàn zhòng xīn* 病变重心.

Dilation: *pǐ* 痞. The term *pǐ* describes a sensation of fullness or a lump. We have used "dilation," meaning expansion or enlargement, as our translation because it seems the most appropriate choice. It does not exclude either aspect of *pǐ*'s meaning, and because it is not used to describe any other specific medical phenomena, it does not have the potential to cause unnecessary confusion.

Pǐ qì 痞气 means *qì* dilation. No shape or form can be felt (there are no space-occupying lesions)—the only symptom is that the patient has subjective feelings of tissue dilation.

Pǐ mǎn 痞满 means dilation fullness. The patient has subjective feelings of being stuffed full.

Pǐ sè 痞塞 means dilation blockage. This term refers to a sensation of blockage.

Pǐ kuài 痞块 means dilation lump. Such lumps occur in conditions such as hepatomegaly, splenomegaly, and liver cancer.

Outpush: *tòu* 透. *Tòu* 透 and *dá* 达 have similar meanings. But in order to make our text easier to read, rather than translating them both as outthrust, we have translated *tòu* as outpush and *dá* as outthrust.

Rash: *bān zhěn* 斑疹. The term *bān zhěn* describes a general condition, not a combination condition, so in order to clarify meaning and make our text easier to read, we have used a general, rather than a combination term.

Reversal: *jué* 厥. This term has two meanings. Firstly, it is the name of a pattern where sudden fainting and possible loss of consciousness is usually followed by gradual spontaneous recovery. Secondly, it is the name of a pattern where the main symptom is cold limbs.

The term *hūn jué* 昏厥 (clouding reversal) specifies the first of these meanings.

The term *zhī jué* 肢厥 (limb reversal) specifies the second of these meanings.

Throughclear: *tōng* 通. *Tōng* means clear through. Since there is no single word in English that carries this meaning we have coined our own, and translated it as "throughclear."

Tongue moss: *shé tāi* 舌苔. *Tāi* means moss or lichen. When applied to the tongue coating, the word "moss" describes not only its appearance, but also the process of its generation. Just as the moss of the external environment is generated by the turbid dampness of earth, the tongue moss is generated by the spleen and stomach *qì* steaming turbid *qì* inside the body.

INDEX

C

D

E

F

M

N

S

T

U

X

Y